D1560526

HOT SEX

OVER 200 THINGS YOU CAN TRY TONIGHT

JAMYE WAXMAN, M.ED.
EMILY MORSE

illustrated by
BENJAMIN WACHENJE

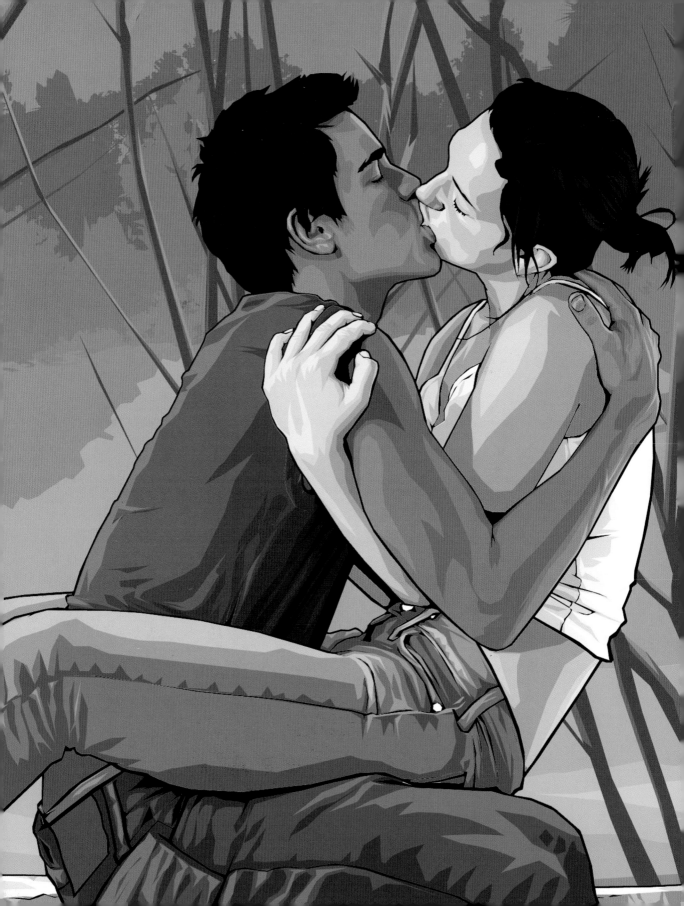

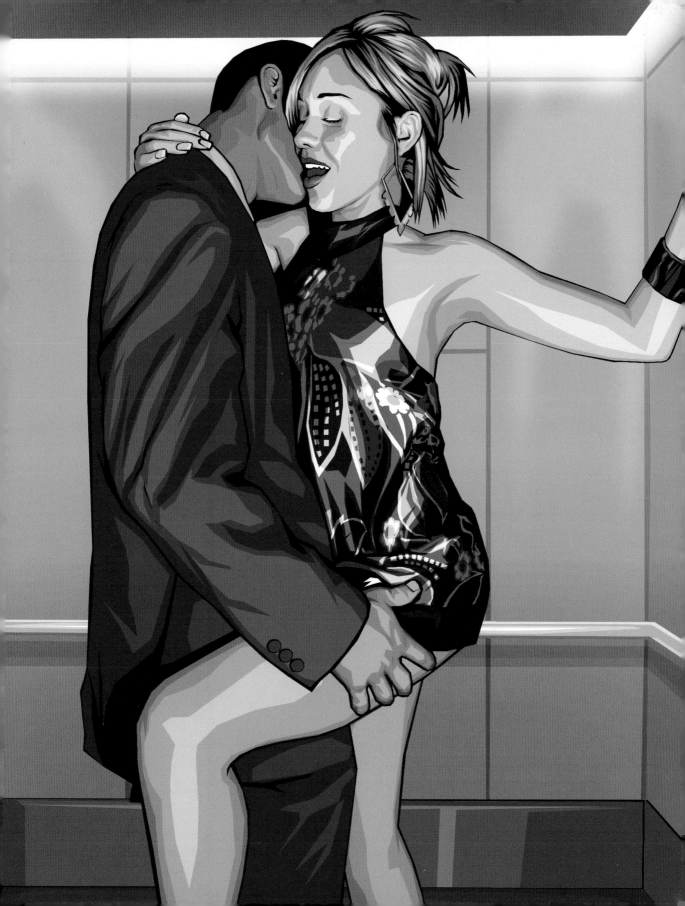

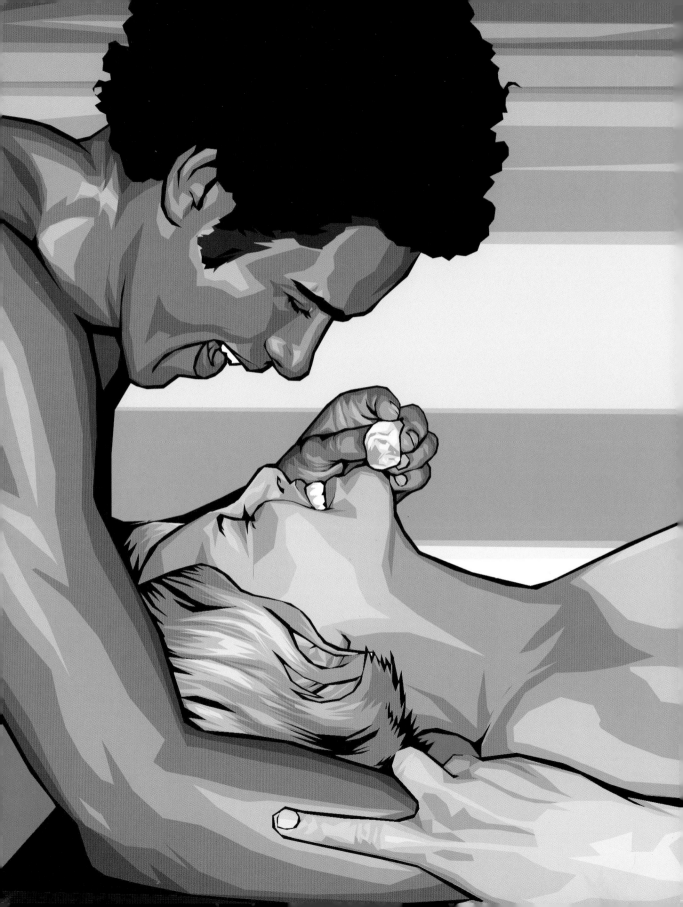

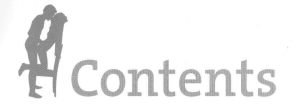

Contents

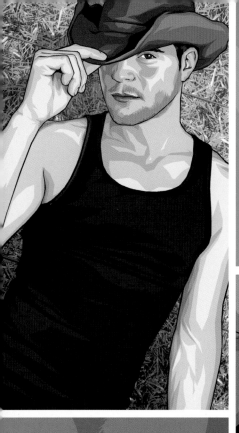

Fun and fearless ideas for role play.

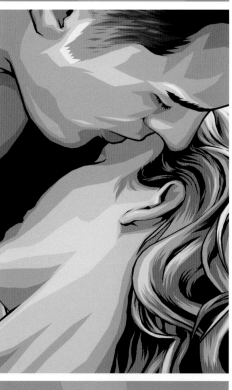

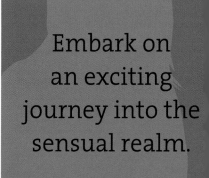

Steamy and sensual ways to build intimacy.

Embark on an exciting journey into the sensual realm.

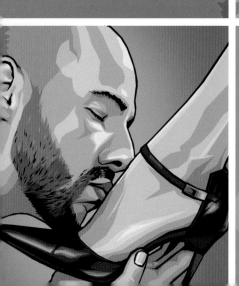

Dress—and undress—for sexy success.

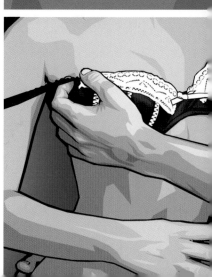

How to make your fantasies come true.

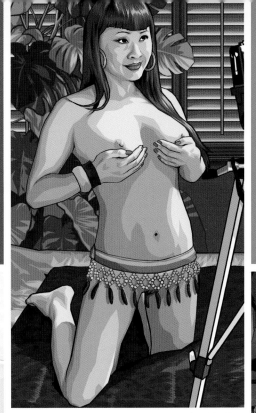

Seductive secrets and saucy games.

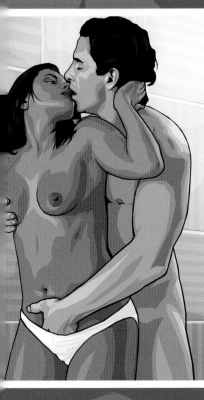

Hands-on hints for teasing and pleasing.

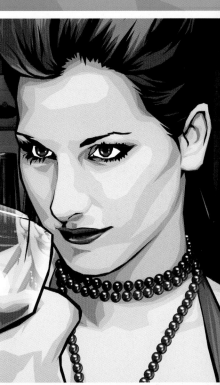

All the most satisfying sex positions.

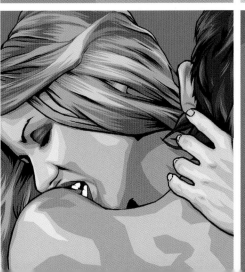

Sweetly sizzling make-out moments.

Jamye

SEX IS . . .

When you think of those two small words, placed side by side, one next to the other, plenty of adjectives run through the mind. Sex is . . . fun. Silly. Explosive. Intimate. Deep. Dynamic. Average. Unexpected. Mind-blowing. Pleasure. Pain. Release. Love.

If you learn only one sex tip from this book, it should be this: enthusiasm. Sex is best with a lot of enthusiasm. There's not one right way to have sex, but if you're not excited to be doing it, it can feel wrong.

What I also love about sex is that it's fluid. It can, and should, change over the course of a lifetime or a relationship. It can be vanilla one day and chocolate the next. You can do it like rabbits or like Kama Sutra masters. You can explore sex with one person or more, of more than one gender.

We use the pronouns "he" and "she" in this book for simplicity's sake. But sex and gender aren't always simple. So, we'd like to take a moment to acknowledge the many ways and partners one person can explore. While you'll see men and women getting down on most of these pages, we're down with you trying anything in this book with any person or people you desire.

My hope is that this book inspires you to make new choices, and to celebrate the choices you've already made. To enjoy what works for you and to laugh about the things that don't. Try to continuously create and explore your sexual self and love the sex you choose to have. Now go to it!

Love,

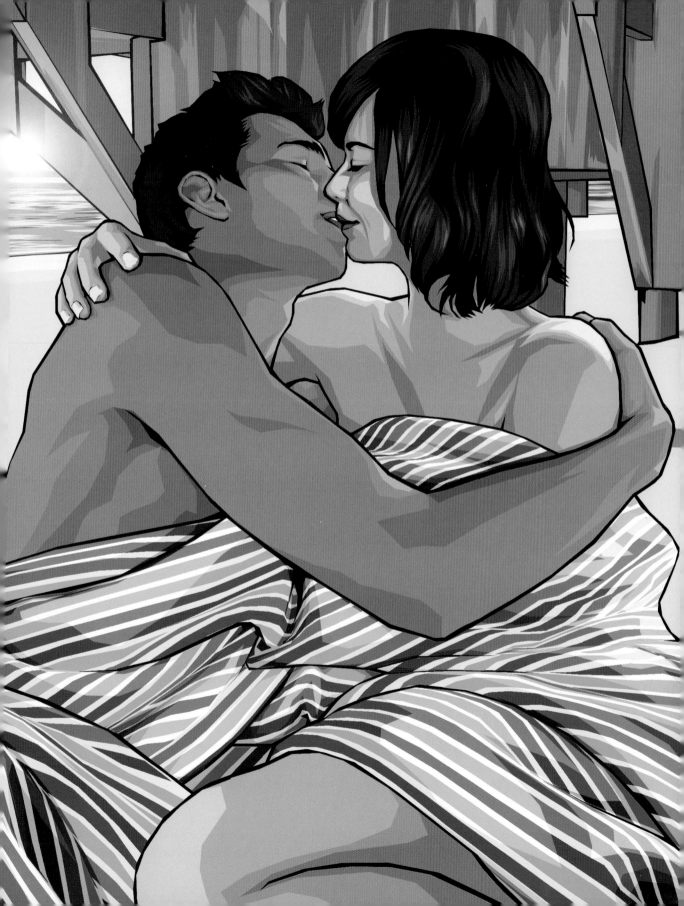

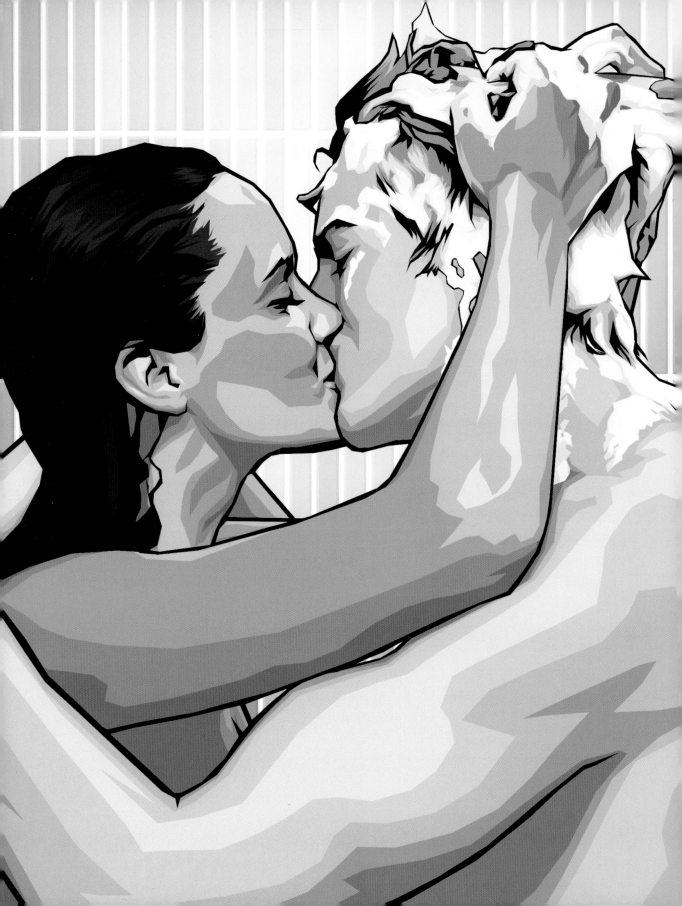

Whenever people say they're having amazing sex, my first thought is, "Good for you." My next is, "What does that mean?" Turns out it means something different for everyone. Amazing sex can be about safety, comfort, ecstasy, orgasm, completion, wholeness, or just some good old-fashioned, toe-curling, gasp-inducing fun.

Even the most sexually aware person can occasionally feel that sex has become routine and it's time to shake things up. The good news is this: you can expand your sexual repertoire with ease. Whether you've been curious about having a threesome, thinking of tying up your partner, or just craving some different takes on the missionary position, this book will get you there.

Communication is a kind of lubrication, and talking to your partner about sex is the best way to keep the excitement and increase the intimacy in your relationship. This book will show you ways to explore and expand your sex life, whether it's a one-night stand or one more night with your lover. These tips work in any bedroom (or backseat) in the world.

Look at these pointers as your erotic road map—or a sexy cookbook full of tantalizing recipes. Read, experiment, and see what works for you.

Remember, you don't have to try everything (it would be amazing if everyone liked every thing in this book—it's a sampler, not a rulebook!). Let the tips inspire you as you flip through the pages, with a partner or by yourself. Try one at a time, a position a week, or two tips a month, and we promise it will shake up, enhance, and supercharge your sex life.

Love,

Emily

TEASE

The secret to a successful tease lies within your ability to hold back and enjoy the journey. Whoever came up with the phrase "the best things come to those who wait" was obviously a devoted fan of teasing. The art of the tease is all about sparking, fanning, and prolonging desire. It can be as simple as a flash of skin, a hint of leg, or a brush of the hand. Whether you're in your living room or out on a date, take steps to create an erotic and fun mood and to get the sexual temperature rising. Where to begin? That's easy—start with your mouth. Words are powerful tools of temptation, so begin by talking about what you'd like to do to each other. Voicing your desires is a huge turn-on and a great way to learn about your partner, and it opens up communication for all the sexy fun that's to come. Then it's time to start touching each other, but do it oh-so-slowly. Stroke and caress each other's bodies, enjoying the anticipation as it builds and builds—the best tease lasts until it makes you feel as if you can't control your desire for a single second longer.

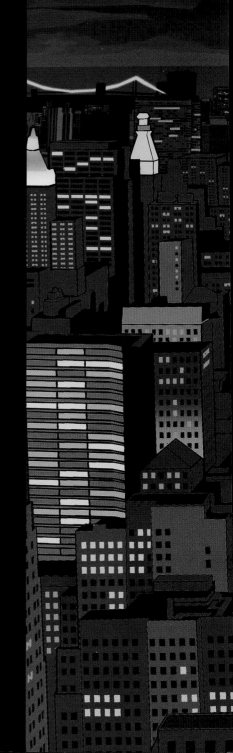

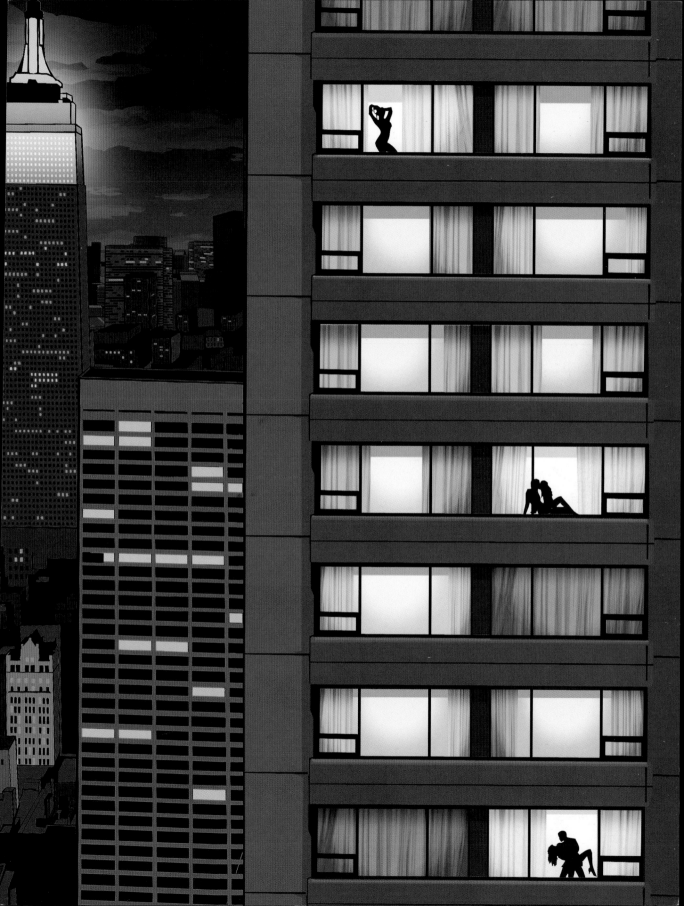

Teasing is the classic way to start up something steamy—and the longer you savor the suspense, the better. The sexiest tease sessions draw on all the senses.

1 START THE SEDUCTION

It all begins with just a touch or a glance. Eye contact is one of the best ways to communicate desire. Watch your lover watching you. Then smile, lick your lips, and raise those brows.

Once you've locked eyes, your touch is another way to express amorous intent. A full-on sensual caress isn't the only way to flirt with your hands; try a light but long-lasting touch as a subtle and nonverbal way to speak volumes. Place your hand on top of your partner's hand, or let your fingers linger on a shoulder.

Your feet are another great way to deepen a sparking connection, especially in public. Play a game of "footsie" when your feet aren't in full view, and act like nothing's going on. Gently rub up against your partner's feet (this works well under a table), then slide your toes from ankle to knee. You can take advantage of the sexy feel of your shoe's leather, or flick it off and use your bare skin or stocking feet. Go as high as you dare, and secretly turn each other on without the rest of the world being turned on to your seduction.

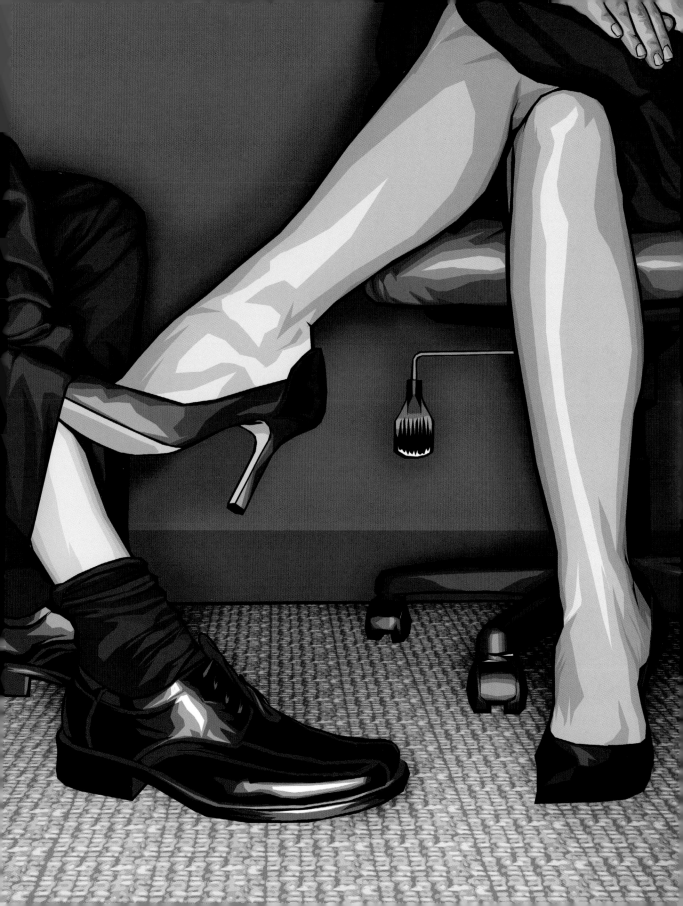

FLIRTING IS FUN

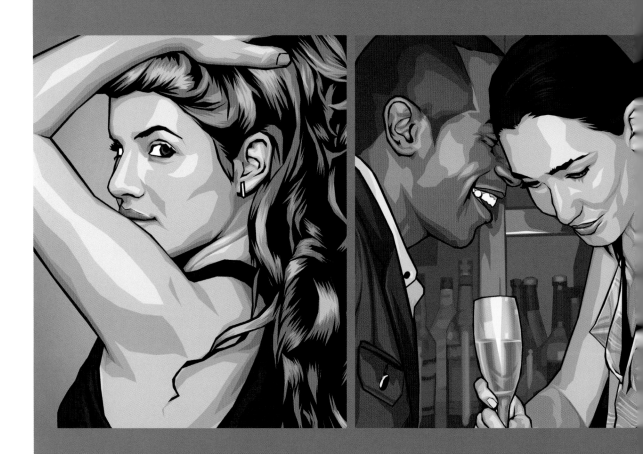

THE MANE EVENT Use your head—or more precisely, your hair—to arouse his interest. Toss those tresses, then run your fingers through them or girlishly twist a curl. Lean in close so he can inhale the clean scent of your shampoo.

PAY ATTENTION You don't have to do or plan anything explicit to flirt with a woman—just use your eyes and words to show her that she's got you riveted. Ask her questions, cleverly riff on her answers, and you'll be well on your way.

TEASE BEFORE GETTING DOWN TO BUSINESS—GET YOUR FLIRT GOING STRONG.

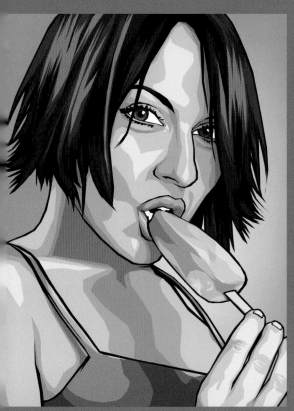

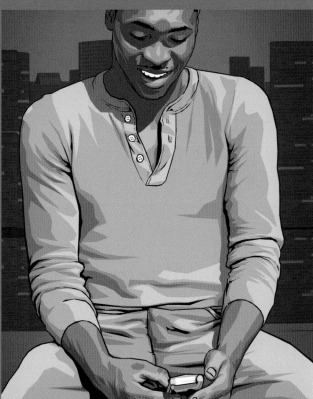

FOOD FOR THOUGHT Watching you eat gets a man thinking about what else you can do with those lips. Play it up with tasty treats that look suggestive, like ice pops, and he'll start thinking about eating you up, too.

SEXTING Sexy texting is a modern way to amp up the passion. Text a naughty fantasy or a hot memory, or talk about what you want to do when you see each other next. Throw in a sexy detail or two, but keep it short and sweet.

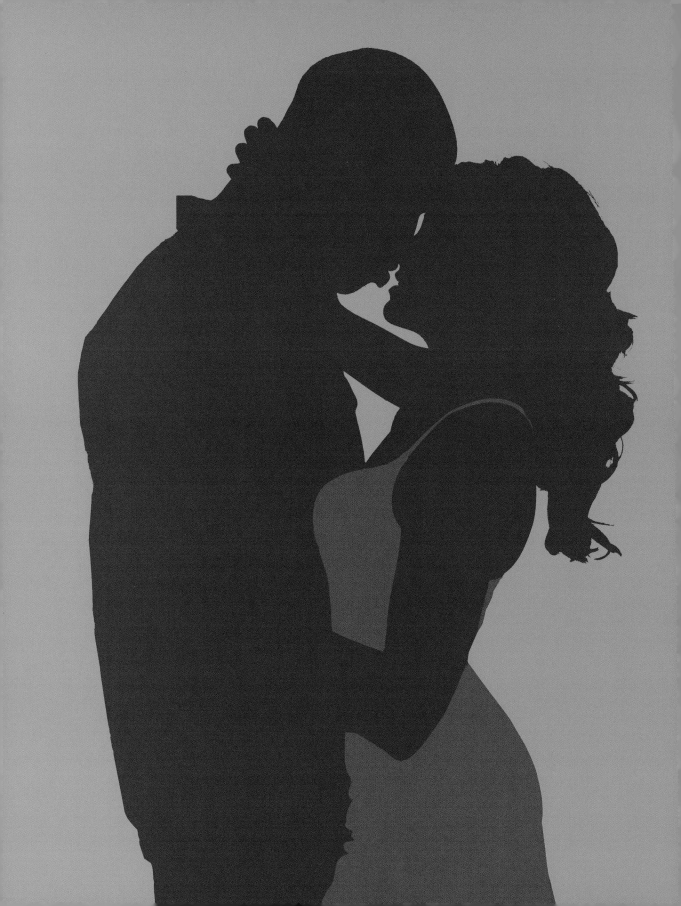

Jamye

"We're not fooling around when we say that making out is really worth your while. Before you seal the deal, do more kissing and clothed caressing, and watch sparks fly."

Emily

"I like the idea of temporarily delaying intercourse so you can focus on kissing and foreplay. Think of foreplay as stretching before a workout—you're simply warming up your body for more action."

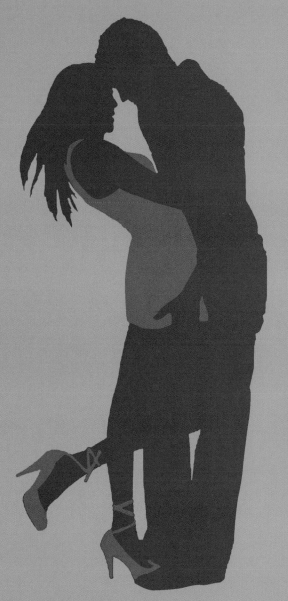

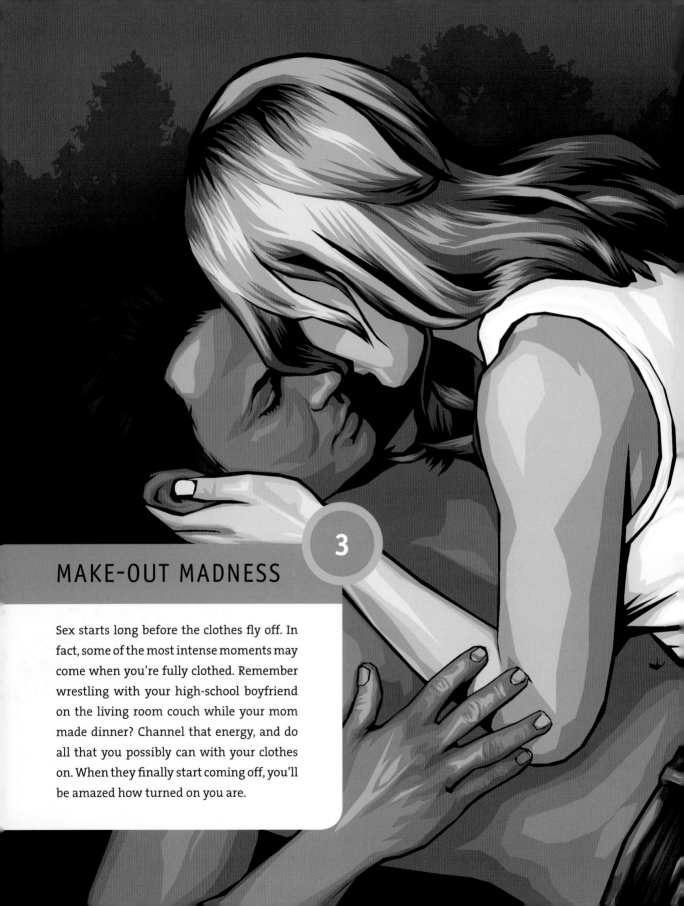

MAKE-OUT MADNESS

3

Sex starts long before the clothes fly off. In fact, some of the most intense moments may come when you're fully clothed. Remember wrestling with your high-school boyfriend on the living room couch while your mom made dinner? Channel that energy, and do all that you possibly can with your clothes on. When they finally start coming off, you'll be amazed how turned on you are.

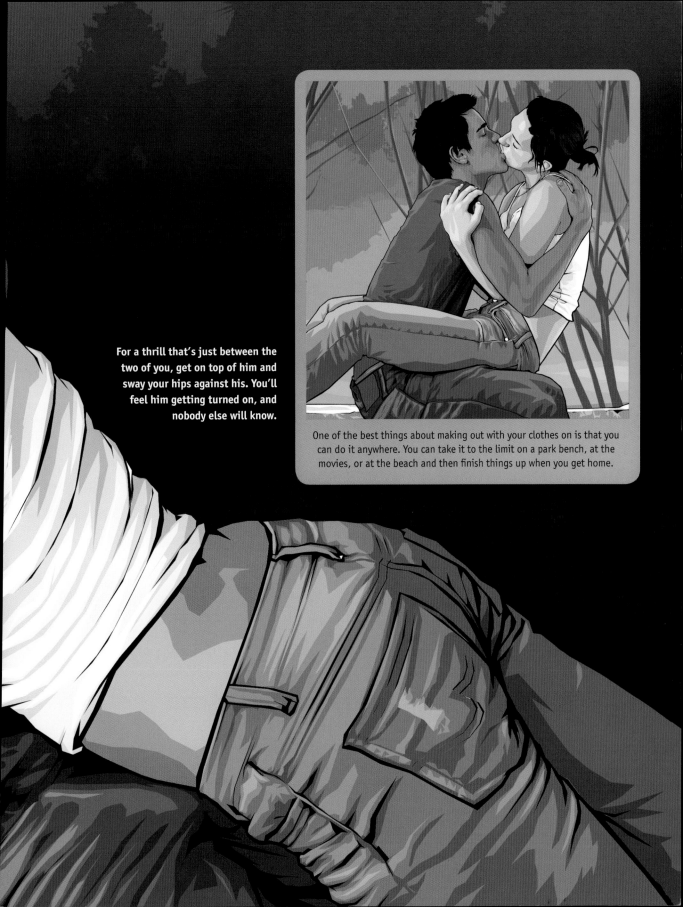

For a thrill that's just between the two of you, get on top of him and sway your hips against his. You'll feel him getting turned on, and nobody else will know.

One of the best things about making out with your clothes on is that you can do it anywhere. You can take it to the limit on a park bench, at the movies, or at the beach and then finish things up when you get home.

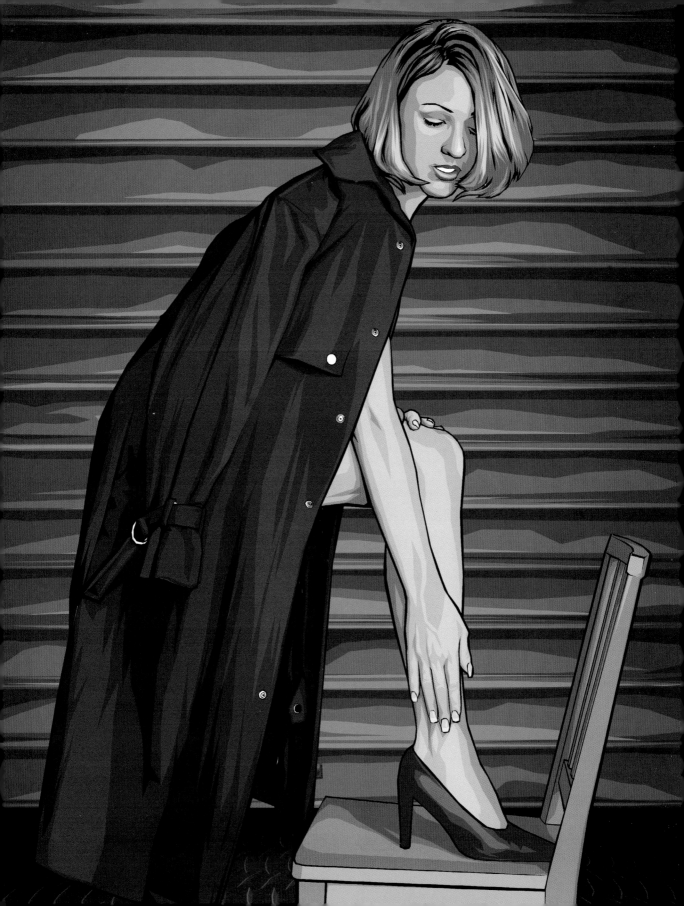

Going all the way in public can get tricky, but a brief glimpse of skin gives him a tantalizing visual treat—plus a preview of the pleasures that lie ahead.

PUT ON A PEEP SHOW 4

Furtive flashes can be a great way to amp up the sexual tension. Be sure to dress for sexy success—any coat that's long enough to be worn as a dress or robe will work: just wear nothing underneath and go for a stroll together. When the spot feels secluded enough, open your coat and give him an eyeful.

For another type of sneak peek, try "accidentally" dropping your fork when you're at a restaurant. When your date goes to pick it up, open your knees so he can see that you're not wearing undies.

Don't underestimate how even a quick glimpse can spark his imagination.

With or without panties, stockings and garter belts add a little ooh-la-la. Or slip on thigh-high fishnets and make sure your honey gets a good look at the sweet spot where fabric meets flesh.

If his attention tends to focus a bit higher on your anatomy, put on a saucy bra or go braless the next time the two of you go out. Wear a loose, scoop-neck shirt so you can bend forward and give him a taste of what's next on the menu.

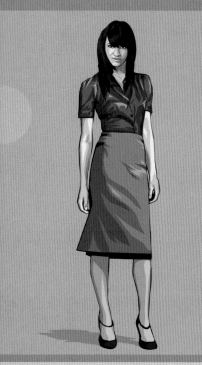
1

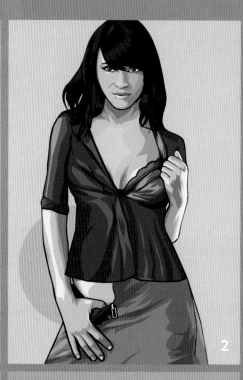
2

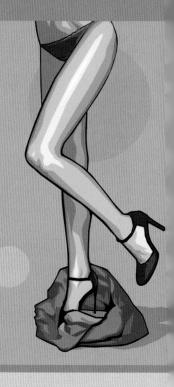

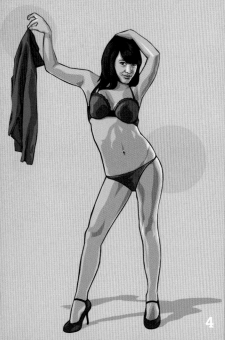
4

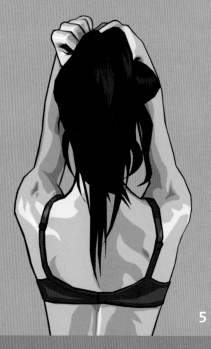
5

{1} Have your partner pick out the clothes he'd like to see you remove. Remember, he thinks you're sexy even if you aren't a supermodel.

{2} Tease him by running your hands over your clothed body.

{3} A skirt can trip up even seasoned strippers. Pin it to the floor with one foot, then step out with the other.

{4} Flatter any figure by saucily cocking your hip to the side.

{5} Play with your hair for sensual appeal. Pull it away from your face, then let it fall in loose, sexy tendrils.

{6} Eye contact enhances mutual attraction. So be sure to watch your partner watching you.

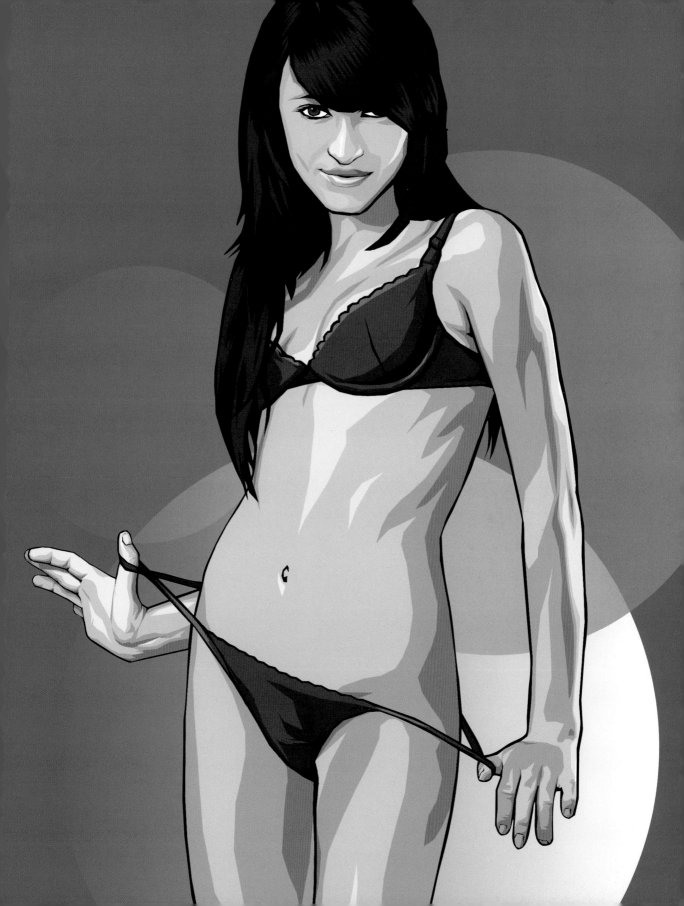

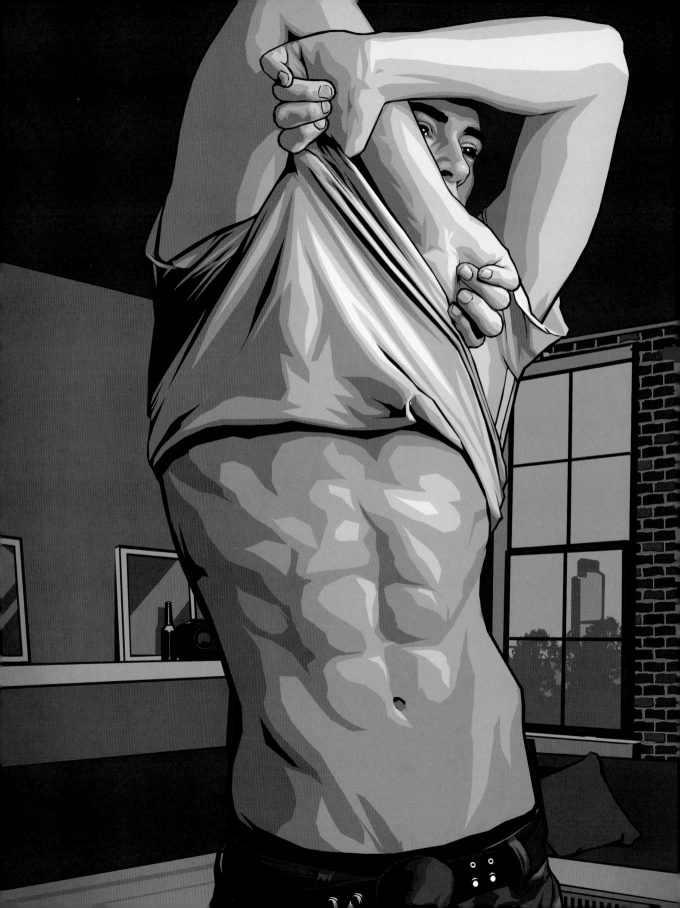

You don't need the body of an athlete or the moves of a Chippendales dancer to put on a hot show for your partner. Just let yourself get caught up in the moment.

ROCK THOSE MANLY MOVES 6

Sexy stripper moves are not just for women—it's time for the guys to strike a pose and dance for their lovers at home. Tear-away pants and thong bikinis are not required, just wear the clothes that she likes to see you in and that make you feel confident—whether that happens to be a power suit or boxer briefs.

Seat your audience of one, put on a sexy song, and stand a few feet in front of her. Tighten up those abs and arch your back slightly so you look your best. Move your hips in time with the music.

Get closer and maintain eye contact as you place one foot in between her legs and circle your hips over her thigh. Bend your knees and grind against her leg. Then turn around and shake your butt. Remove your clothing slowly, sliding your hands all over your body.

To heighten the sexual tension, follow the rules of a strip club: she can look, but she can't touch. Get as close as you can without actually making contact with her (or brush across her skin briefly), and she'll likely insist on a steamy encore.

Emily

"Remember, kisses aren't just for the lips. Try planting kisses on the often-neglected neck, ears, nose, eyelids, fingers—you get the picture. Sometimes a kiss in an unexpected place is just what these other erogenous zones ordered."

Jamye

"When it comes to kissing, it definitely takes some time to find the right rhythm. Play follow-the-leader, and have one person lead the kiss, while the other person follows their moves. Then switch!"

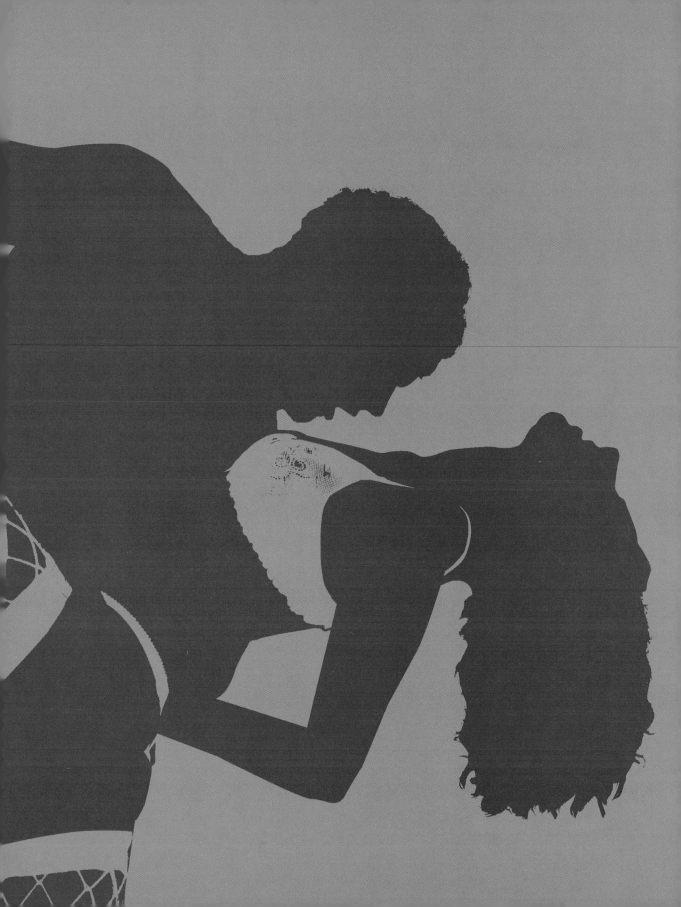

MAKE THE MOST OF YOUR MOUTH

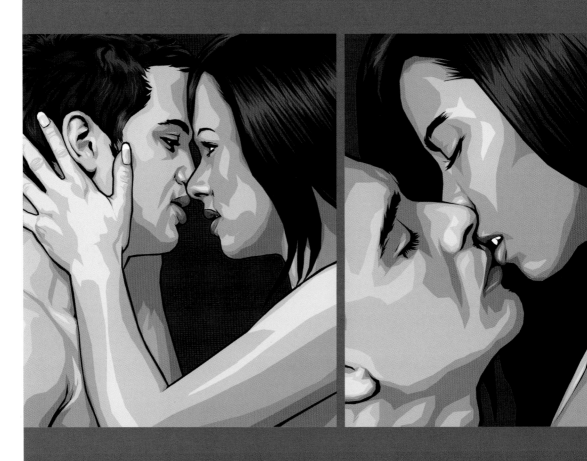

1 **GAZE** We can't emphasize this point enough—eye contact adds heat to intimate interactions. Look long, and gaze deeply into each other's pupils. Guiding your partner's face in toward yours is a sexy, take-charge move.

2 **KISS** Kissing can be done in many ways, so try out a range of techniques. Go soft and tentative with your lips barely brushing one another. Next, try long, deep kisses with lots of tongue. Nibble gently on the lower lip.

SEX IS A BANQUET—FEEL FREE TO LICK, NIBBLE, AND BITE ALL YOU WANT.

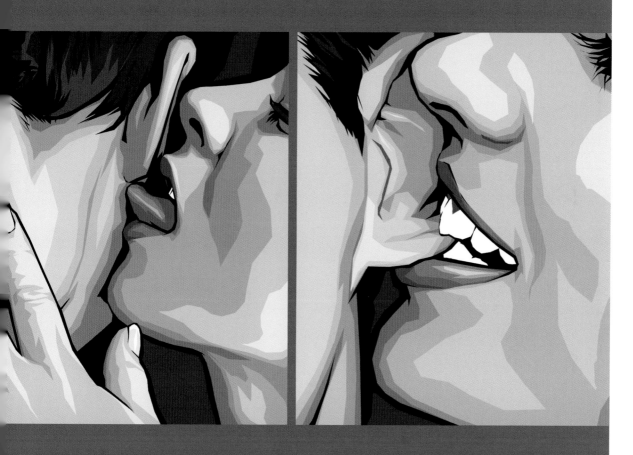

3 **LICK** To raise the temperature, use that tongue. For playful goodness, visit the neck and ears as well as some often-ignored erogenous zones—like the bends in the arms, behind the knees and between fingers and toes.

4 **BITE** Don't be afraid to use your teeth to give your partner added pleasure (and a sexy hint of pain). Light bites are a good way to start. Begin gently with the ears and the neck. If your partner enjoys it, build up to harder pressure.

What's sexier than a half-naked man or woman? Enjoy the view—and the sizzling sense of anticipation—as you start to get hot, heavy, and excited to go all the way.

8 LINGER IN YOUR LINGERIE

The temperature is rising, and by now you're getting hot and heavy. The natural impulse is to just rip each other's clothes off and go wild. Instead, keep the tension building. Once you take it all off, there's only one thing left to do. Making the most of the delicious moment just before sex will bring your arousal levels to a fever pitch. Humans are visual creatures, so take a moment to appreciate how your partner looks when nearly naked. Run your fingers over erogenous zones, letting the texture of the cloth amplify your touch. Slide your fingers under waistbands and straps—but not too far.

Undergarments create just the right amount of obstacle to intercourse (unless of course you just slide them to the side and have sex without getting fully undressed, which can be a really hot move). Before you remove those last little pieces of fabric, kiss and touch everywhere else. Build up the excitement with eye contact and erotic talk until you can't stand it any longer and absolutely must move on to the main event.

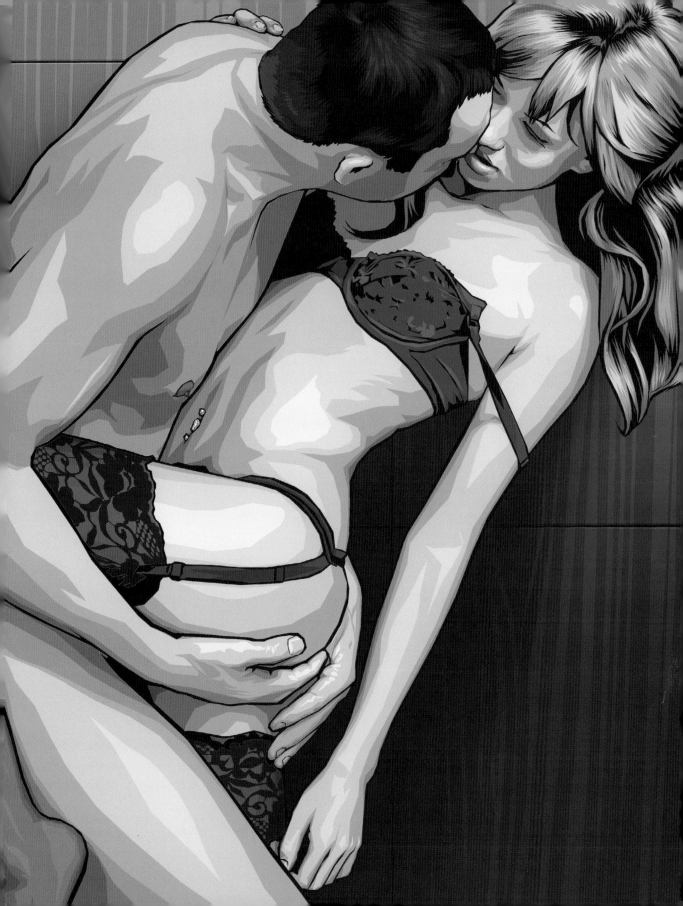

SKIN-ON-SKIN SENSATIONS

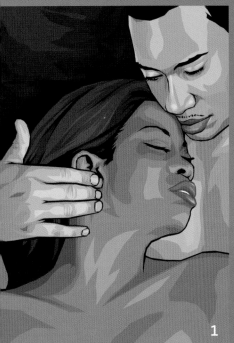

1

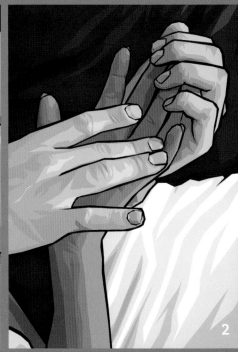

2

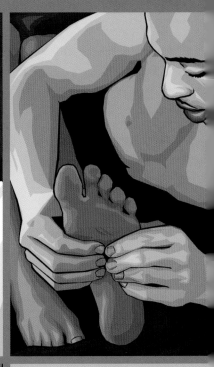

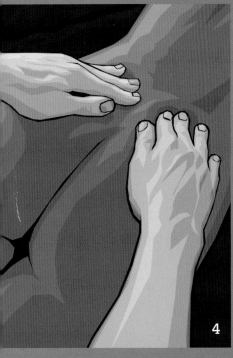

4

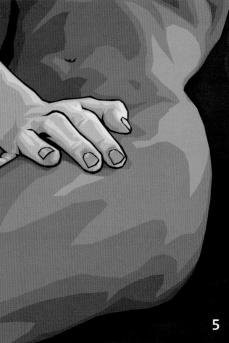

5

{1} The ears are sensitive to touch and immensely sensual. Trace the lobes, then gently massage the tips and the area behind the ears.

{2} Reach for the hands and apply pressure in sweeping arcs over the palms, then work between the fingers.

{3} Slather on massage lotion and work the feet from heel to toe. Tip: the back of the foot above the heel is a supersweet spot.

{4} When massaged, the dimples in the lower back can release erotic energy. Try a circular motion.

{5} Brush up the inner thigh from the knee to just under the hip with long, sweeping strokes.

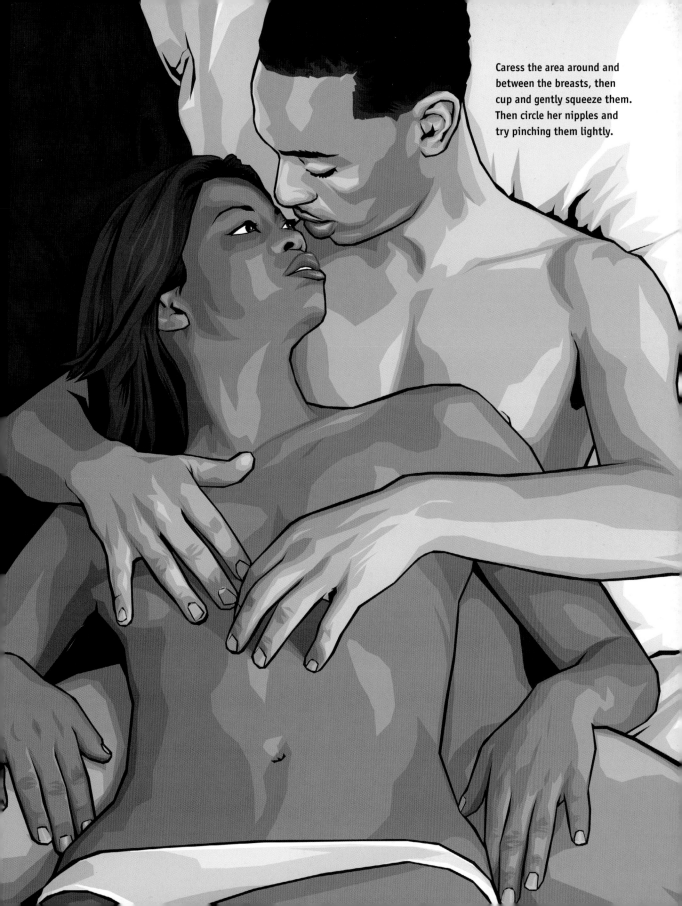

Caress the area around and
between the breasts, then
cup and gently squeeze them.
Then circle her nipples and
try pinching them lightly.

DRESSING DOWN

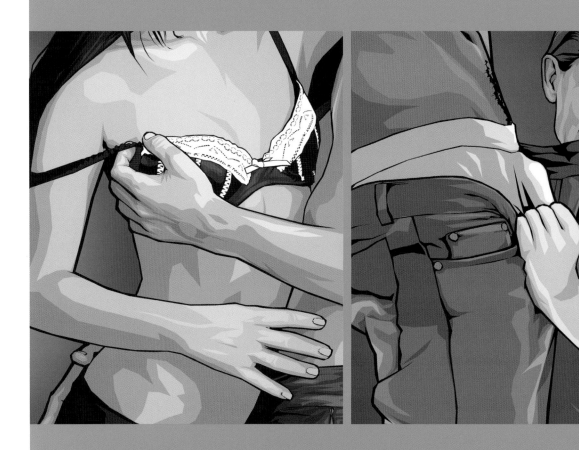

SLOW HANDS Take your time removing her bra. Before you start, look into her eyes and tell her how hot she is. Slowly slide the straps down while caressing her shoulders. Can't figure out the clasp? She's likely going to be eager to help.

ANIMAL INSTINCTS When undressing your partner, try channeling your wild side. Sure, hands are fine for disrobing, but why not (carefully!) use your teeth? Tearing at his jeans like a tiger may turn your bedroom into a wild kingdom.

A LITTLE AUDIENCE PARTICIPATION CAN MAKE A STRIPTEASE EVEN HOTTER.

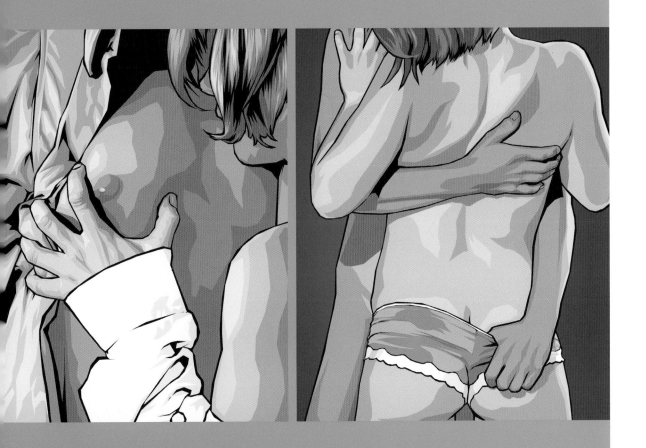

(UN)BUTTONED DOWN If his shirt is one that slips over his head, ask him to raise his arms and playfully tug it off. If it has buttons, undo them one at a time and kiss or lick each new inch of torso as it's exposed. Tease his nipples just a bit.

PANTY RAID Use your fingertips to trace the outline of her privates through the thin fabric of her underwear. Place a finger or two under the waistband, but don't go too far down. Once she starts to squirm, slowly slide those panties off.

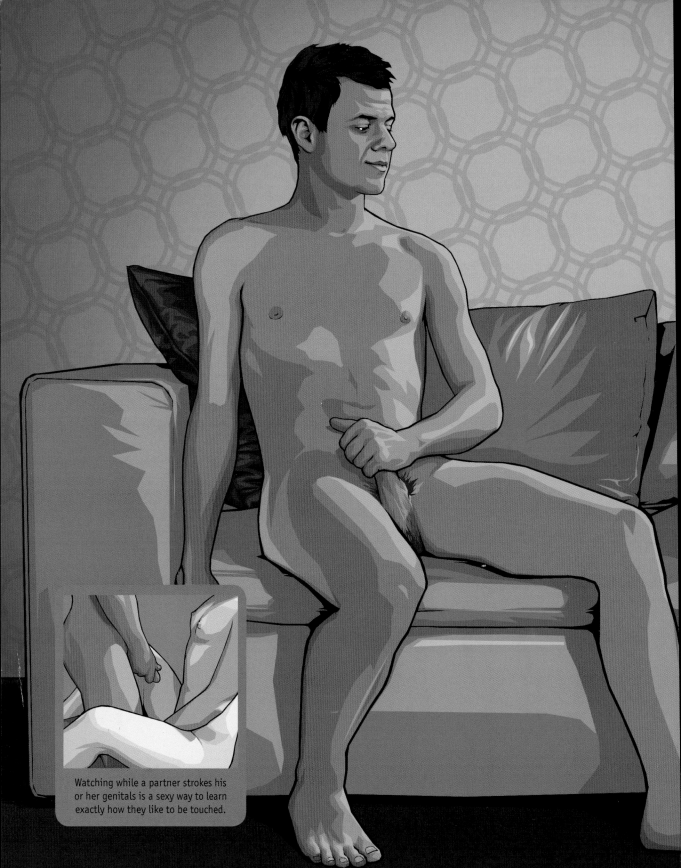

Watching while a partner strokes his or her genitals is a sexy way to learn exactly how they like to be touched.

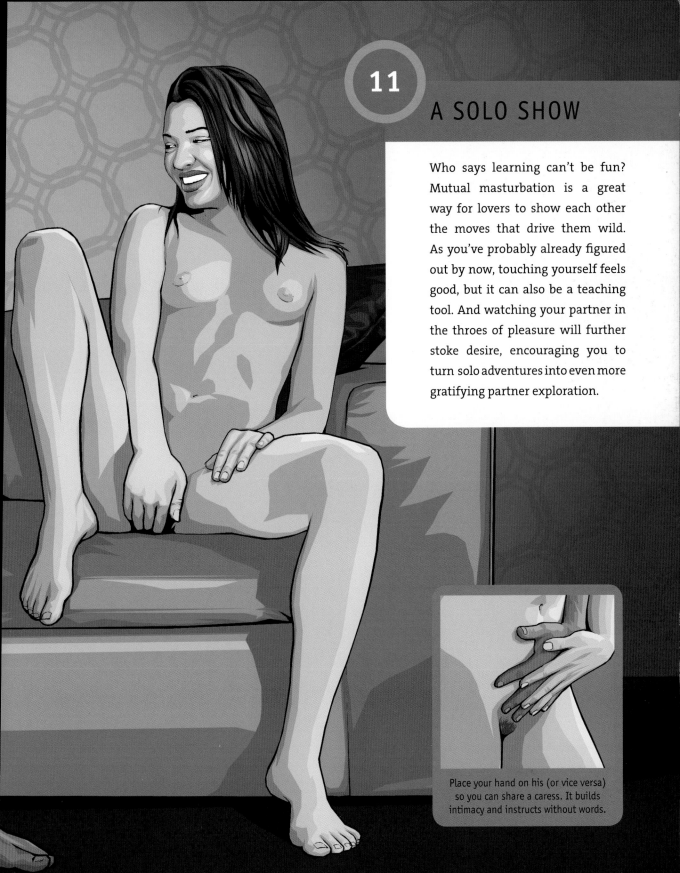

A SOLO SHOW

Who says learning can't be fun? Mutual masturbation is a great way for lovers to show each other the moves that drive them wild. As you've probably already figured out by now, touching yourself feels good, but it can also be a teaching tool. And watching your partner in the throes of pleasure will further stoke desire, encouraging you to turn solo adventures into even more gratifying partner exploration.

Place your hand on his (or vice versa) so you can share a caress. It builds intimacy and instructs without words.

Emily

"When you focus on the senses, even one at a time, you're on your way to great sex. Try targeting the area near a hot zone. For example, trace your fingers around nipples or along the inner thighs. Stimulating nerve endings that radiate outward from the hot spots will lead to more thrilling sensations."

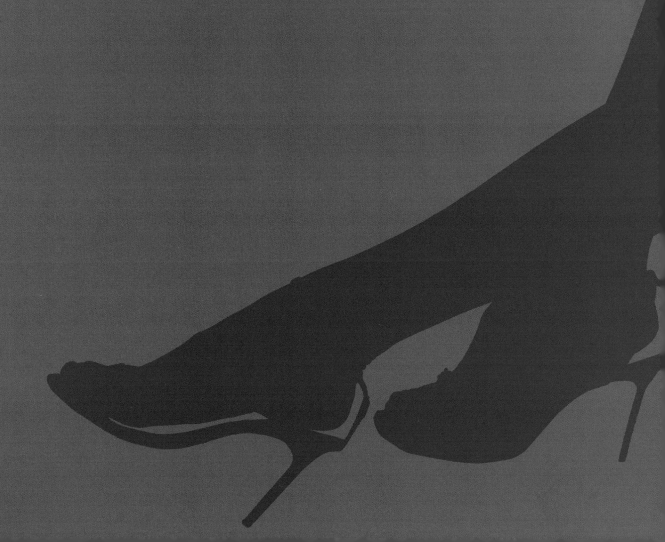

Jamye

"Try getting kinky in your kitchen. Place a tablecloth down on a counter or tabletop, then open the freezer and tease your lover with ice cubes. Grab a stick of butter and get your baby all slippery. Take a wooden spoon and use it for light love taps. Get creative when it comes to stirring up the senses."

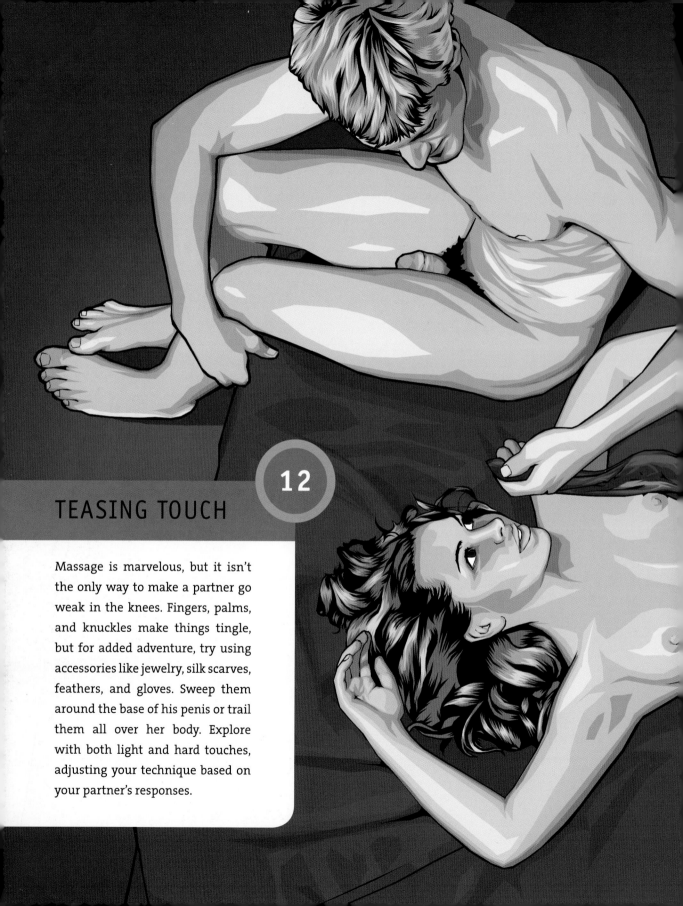

TEASING TOUCH

Massage is marvelous, but it isn't the only way to make a partner go weak in the knees. Fingers, palms, and knuckles make things tingle, but for added adventure, try using accessories like jewelry, silk scarves, feathers, and gloves. Sweep them around the base of his penis or trail them all over her body. Explore with both light and hard touches, adjusting your technique based on your partner's responses.

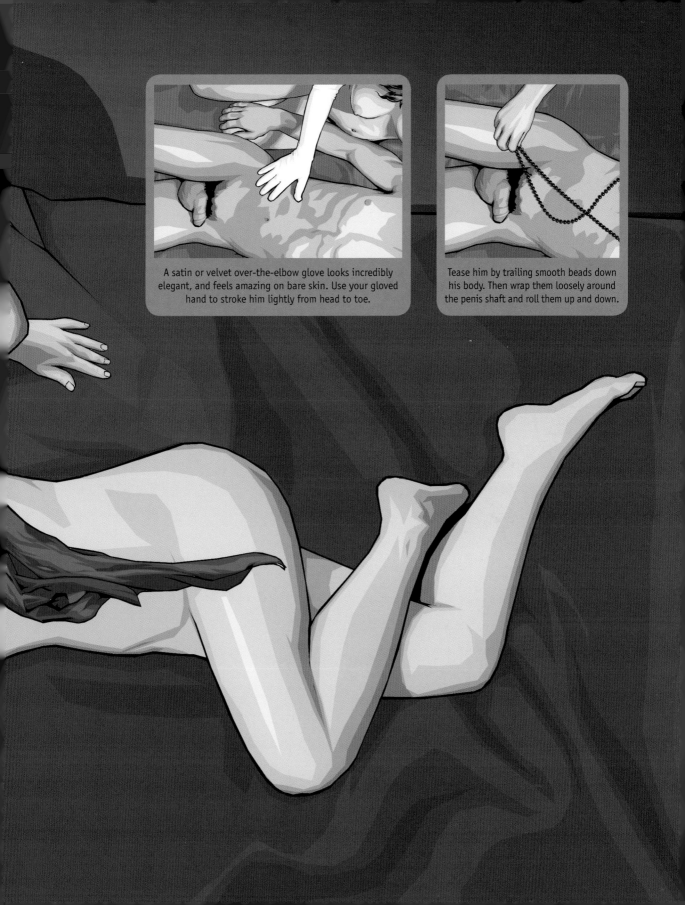

A satin or velvet over-the-elbow glove looks incredibly elegant, and feels amazing on bare skin. Use your gloved hand to stroke him lightly from head to toe.

Tease him by trailing smooth beads down his body. Then wrap them loosely around the penis shaft and roll them up and down.

SURPRISING SENSATIONS

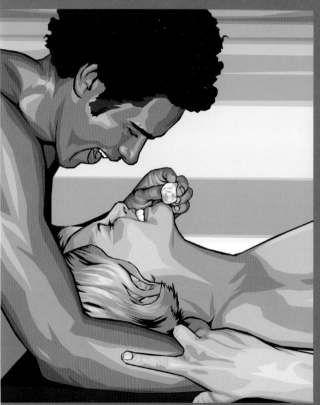
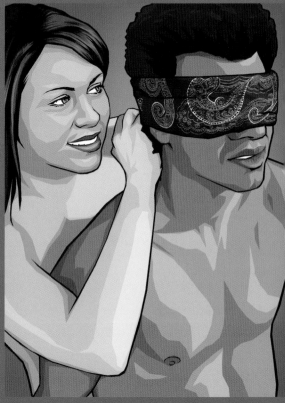

ICE, ICE BABY When you want to give someone a delicious chill, take a cube of ice and slide it over the neck, nipples, and belly. Or keep a piece in your mouth as you let your lips explore your partner's contours and erogenous areas.

BLINDERS ON When you remove one sense, you heighten the others. Use a scarf or a necktie to cover your partner's eyes and show him some love. The less he can see, the more he can feel. So send his nerve endings into overdrive.

BE IT HOT OR COLD, FINGERS OR FEATHERS, THE UNEXPECTED CAN BE OH-SO-SEXY.

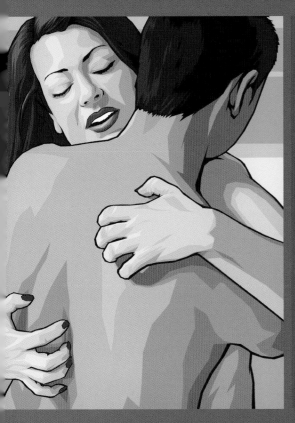

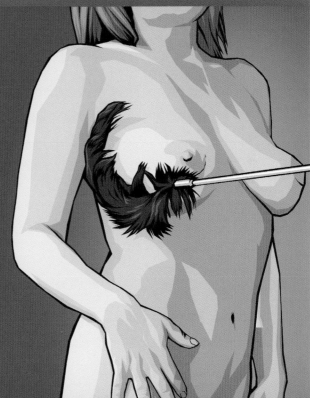

MAKE YOUR MARK Running your nails down your partner's body leaves some sexy evidence and adds a little kink. Start slowly—some people only enjoy a light scratch, others a bit more. An eye-catching manicure adds to the visuals.

FEATHERED FRIENDS You can choose a big ostrich feather or a gaudy peacock plume—either way, feathers are a great way to tickle and tease. The sensation is subtle yet significant and, when paired with a blindfold, especially intriguing.

PLAY

It's true—couples that play together stay together. Whether it's seductively feeding each other fruit as part of a tropical fantasy, touching familiar body parts in a more unexpected way (foot massage, anyone?), or dressing up in sexy costumes, novelty is a great aphrodisiac, and play is a core element of sexy good times. Laughing and joking around together actually stimulate "feel good" brain chemicals that can intensify your connection. So, don't forget to giggle together. Have a pillow fight. Use sex toys. Add props. Experiment with power dynamics. Lavish attention on each other with your hands and mouths, exploring each other's bodies without necessarily moving along to intercourse. Remember, different sensations are just as exciting even if they don't bring you to orgasm. Make special dates that are just for play when you use these tips to titillate and entice each other in brand-new ways. Most importantly, don't be afraid to take the plunge and push your boundaries in the name of fun.

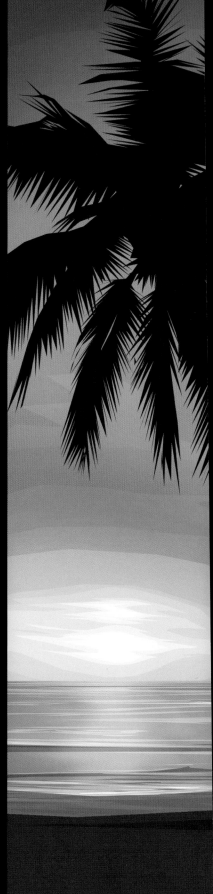

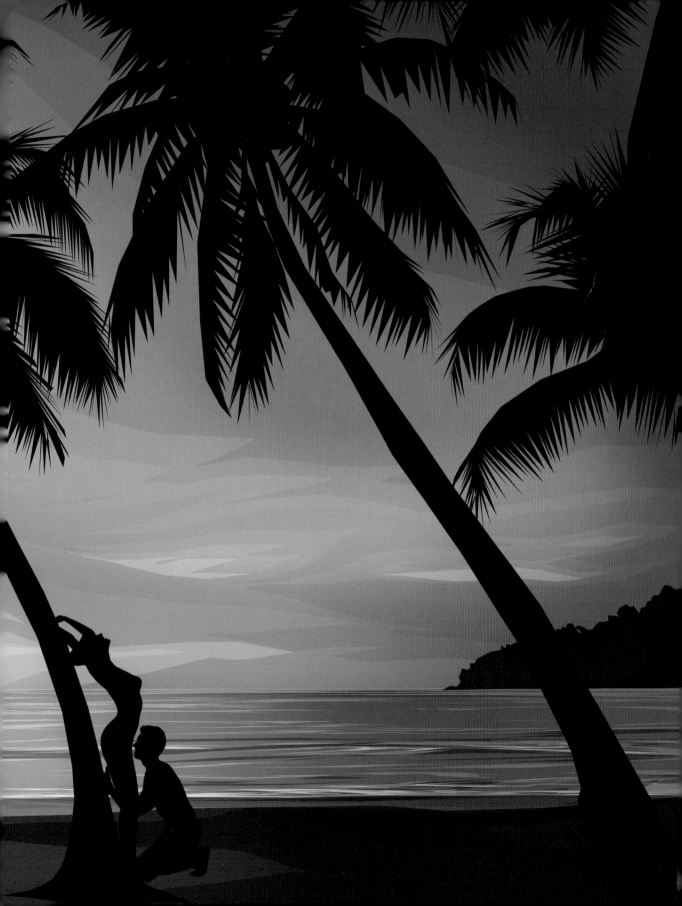

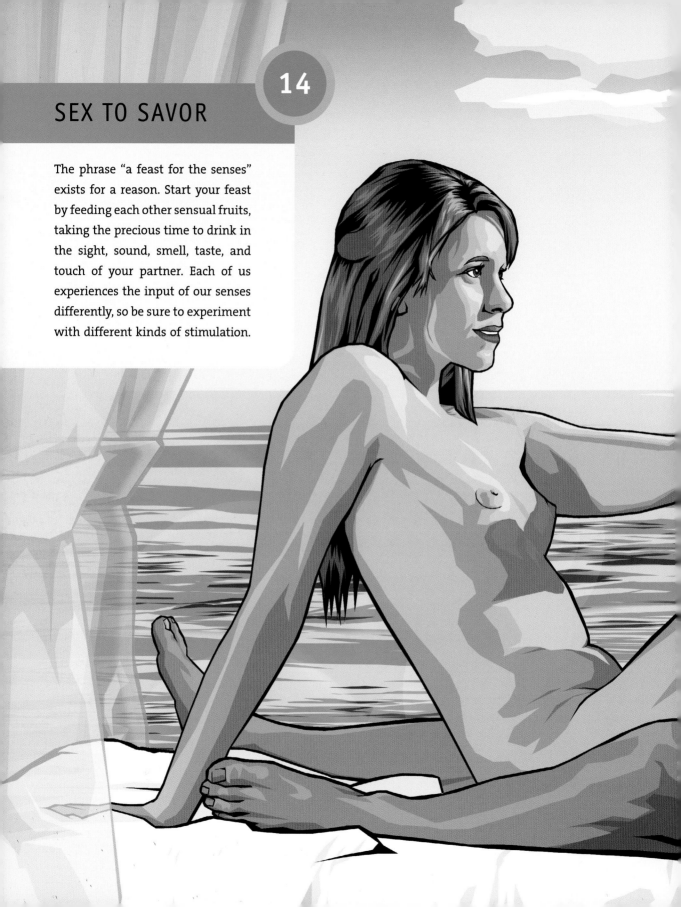

14

SEX TO SAVOR

The phrase "a feast for the senses" exists for a reason. Start your feast by feeding each other sensual fruits, taking the precious time to drink in the sight, sound, smell, taste, and touch of your partner. Each of us experiences the input of our senses differently, so be sure to experiment with different kinds of stimulation.

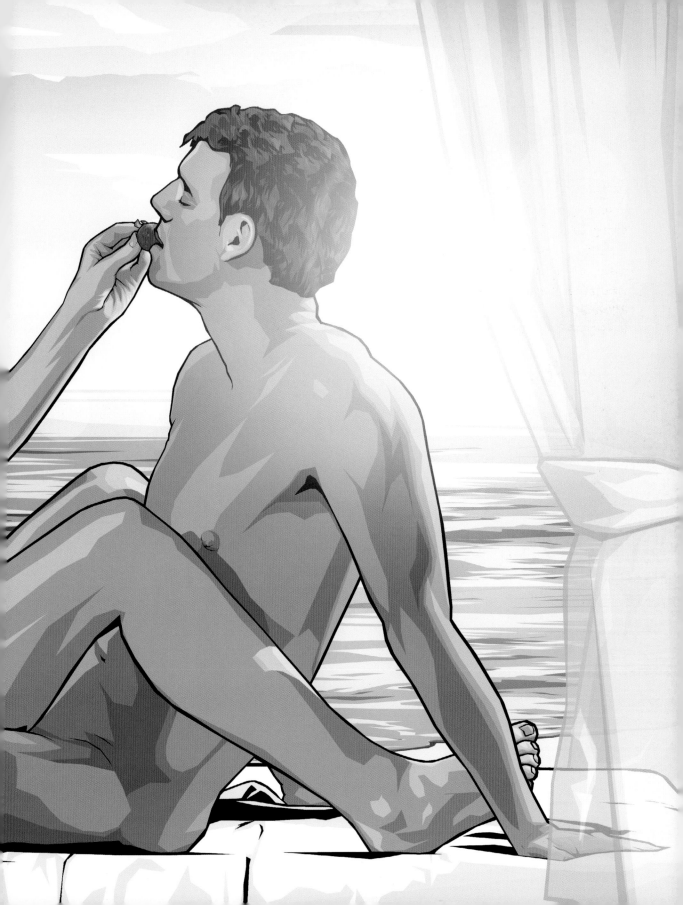

15

A FEAST FOR THE SENSES

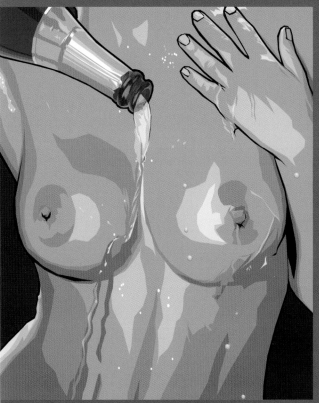 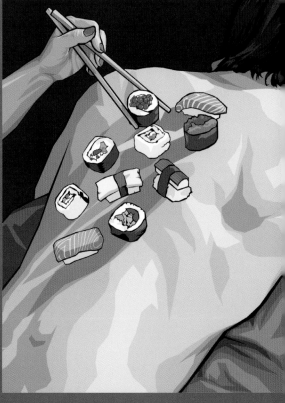

FUN AND FIZZY If you're a big fan of bubbly, pamper your sweetheart with a fizzy champagne bath. Pour a splash on her breasts and lap it up, or take a sip and slowly release it as you move your mouth up his shaft during oral sex.

SERVICE WITH A SMILE Sushi, fruit, or cheese and crackers all taste better when served on a hot human platter. Whether you use chopsticks or your tongue and fingers as utensils, have your fill of both the treats and the server.

SOMETIMES IT'S FUN TO PLAY WITH YOUR FOOD—AND YOUR PARTNER.

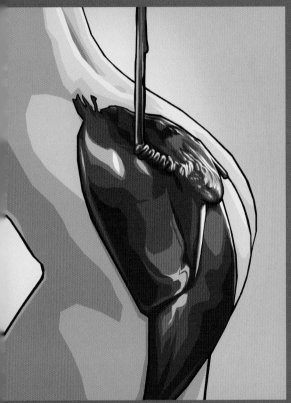 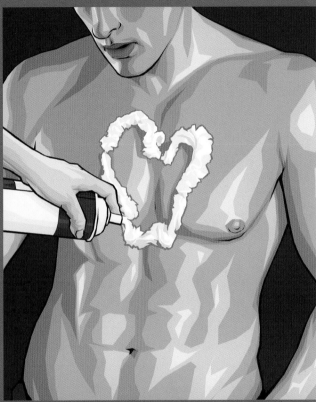

STICKY FINGERS Drizzle some naughty words onto your partner's body with chocolate syrup or honey, then erase them with your tongue. Be very careful never to get any food or sugary syrups inside—keep this an external treat.

CREAMY DREAMS Grab some whipped topping and adorn your lover's body. Most creamy concoctions contain oil, so if you use them below his belt, lick it all off before you put on a condom (again, never put anything sugary in a woman).

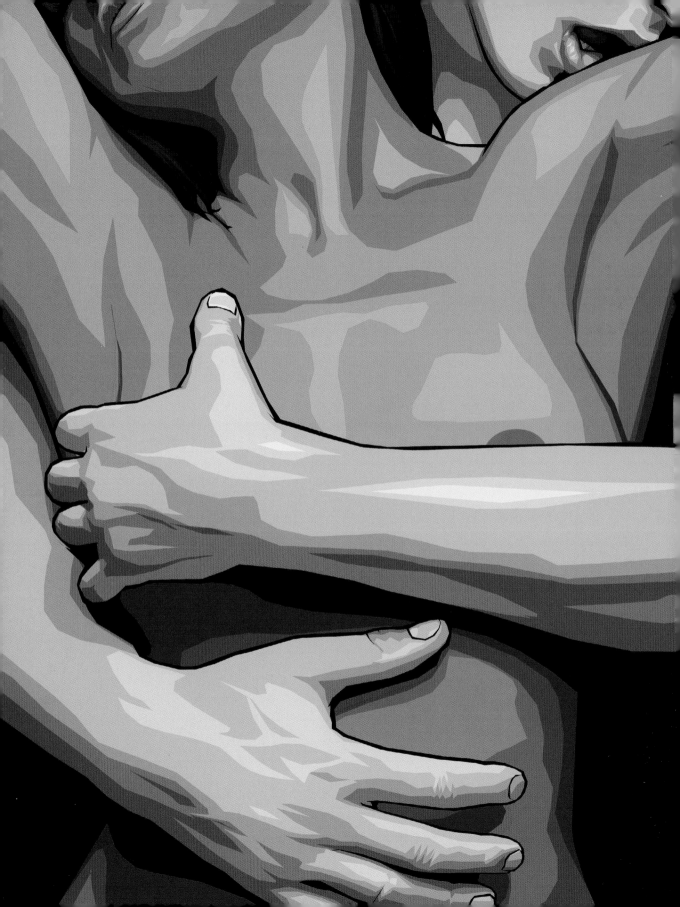

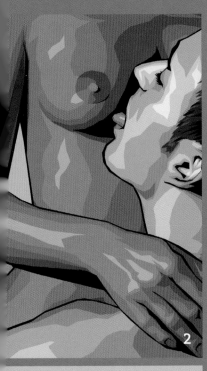

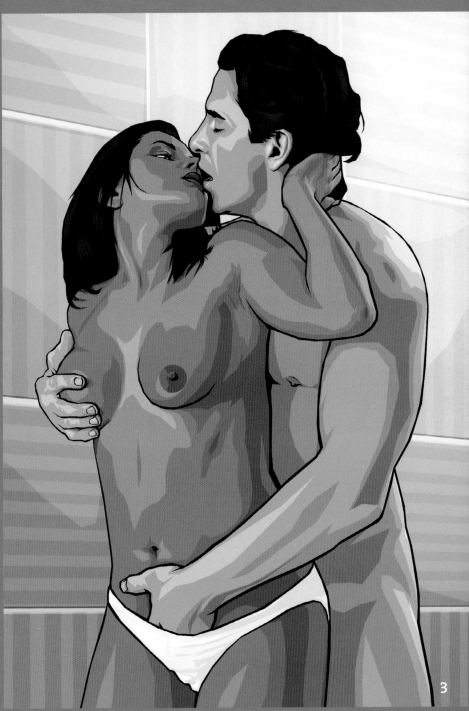

{1} Most men love playing with breasts—and some enjoy having their own chests and nipples teased and stroked. Either way, start off light before trying firmer types of touch.

{2} Flick nipples gently with your tongue, suck lightly, then try out some stronger suction or even a gentle nibble. Use your mouth or fingers to trace around the areola. Intensify the sensation by teasing one nipple with your hand while licking or sucking the other.

{3} Cup her breasts in your hands and massage the sides of each with your thumbs. Place your flattened palm over her nipples and areolas and perform a circular massage.

Instead of going straight for her hot spots, take time to tantalize. Let her groans of pleasure guide you as you try out a range of speeds and intensities.

17 HAND HER SOME PLEASURE

Cup your hand over her entire pubic area, then slowly brush your fingers up and down her inner and outer lips. Keep one finger on each side of her outer lips, then slide your middle finger along the inner lips as you continue to stroke her. Next, focus on her clitoris, gently squeezing the hood between two fingers and lightly moving them up and down.

Next, move your fingers in a clockwise circle around her clitoris, stopping at each "hour" on the clock. Slowly make your way inside of her, asking if and when she'd like you to. You don't have to go deep—the first one-third of the vagina is the most sensitive.

Curve your fingers toward her belly button to find the G-spot. Not all women enjoy this kind of stimulation, so ask before you experiment too much.

Return to the clitoris, as that's how most women climax. Make circles on and around it, then tap it and rub its base as you read the feedback from her body. If she starts getting close to orgasm, keep your motions steady until she climaxes.

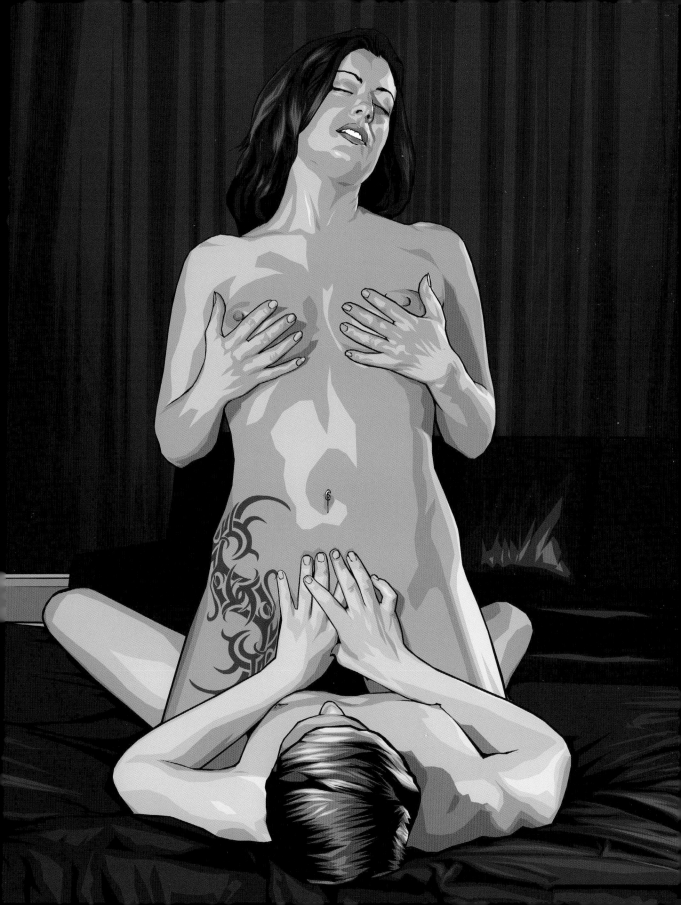

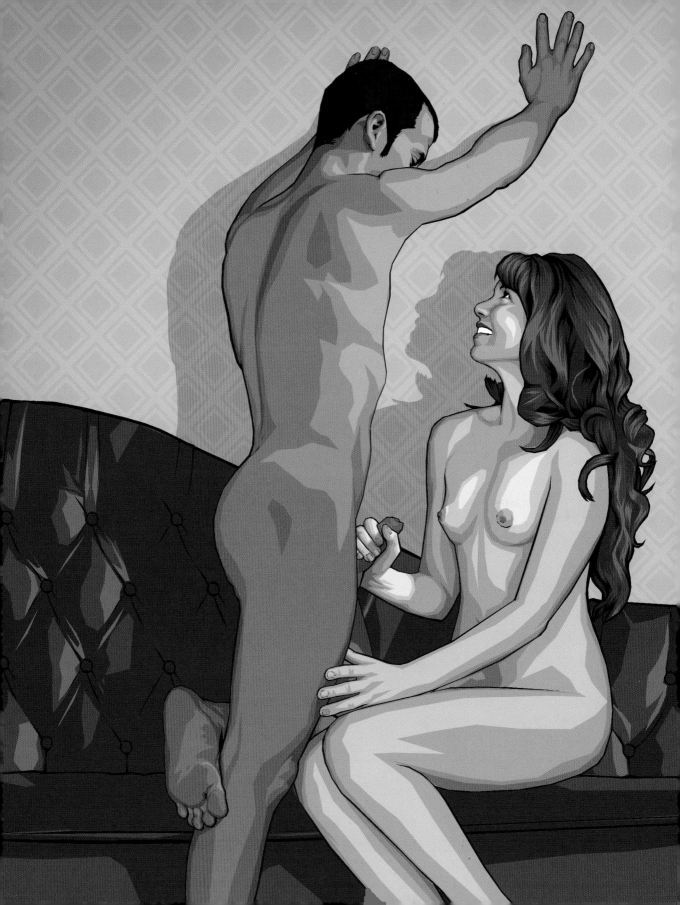

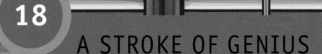

18

A STROKE OF GENIUS

Don't wait until he's fully erect to start stroking his penis. Your touch can help get him in the mood. Some men prefer more attention to the head; others like the focus to be on the shaft. While it's good to vary the stimulation, spend the most time on the areas of his penis that give him the most pleasure. Don't be shy about asking him what feels best.

Try gripping the base with one hand while you slowly move the other up and down, switching occasionally to vary the sensation. In addition to stroking with your whole hand, try making a circle with your thumb and pointer fingers and stroking it up and down, twisting your wrist from side to side. Or stroke straight up and down, but give a little extra twist right at the frenulum, the "V" shape on the underside of his shaft, which is the most sensitive part of the head for many men. A combo of passion, enthusiasm, and visual stimulation add up to a superhot hand job.

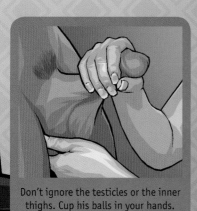

Don't ignore the testicles or the inner thighs. Cup his balls in your hands.

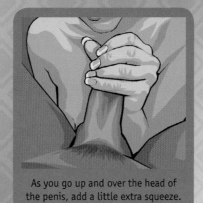

As you go up and over the head of the penis, add a little extra squeeze.

There's no one right way to do it, or even one best angle. Try stroking him while standing behind him so that he can feel your touch from the same angle he does when he pleasures himself—with your body pressed up against him. The penis is the star of this show, but explore other hot spots—whether that means his testicles, perineum (the skin between the scrotum and anus), or prostate. Try firm pressure on the perineum to stimulate the prostate externally.

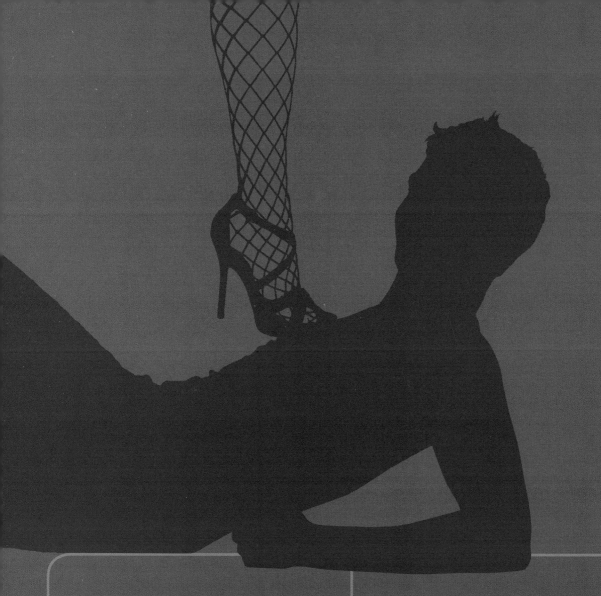

FIVE COMMON MALE SEXUAL FANTASIES

- Finding new ways to please you
- Being dominated
- Threesome sex
- Anal sex
- Watching his partner masturbate

FIVE COMMON FEMALE SEXUAL FANTASIES

- Sex in public
- Group sex
- Being taken by force
- Sex with strangers
- Sex with another woman

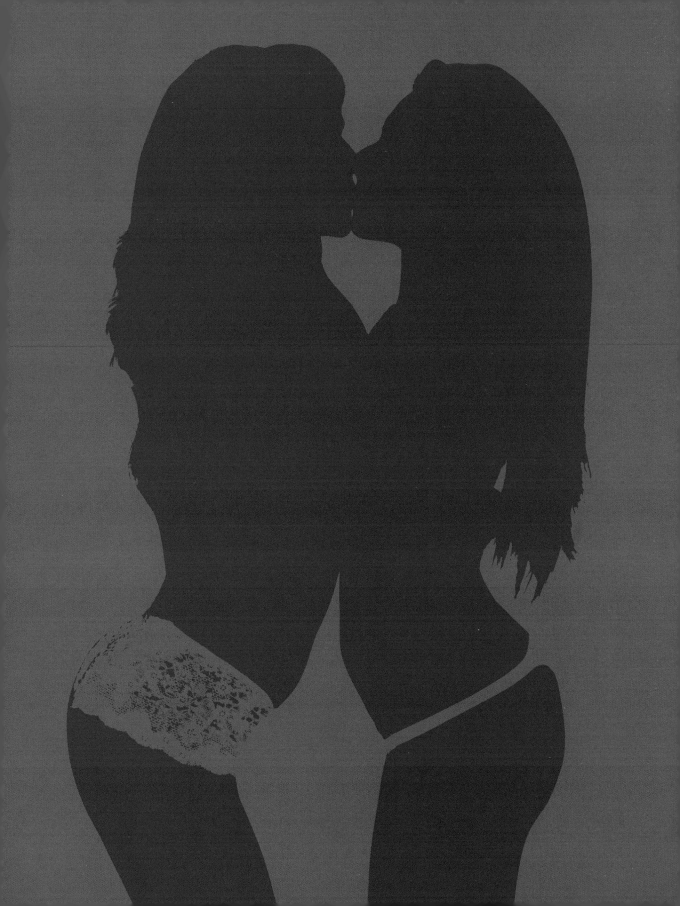

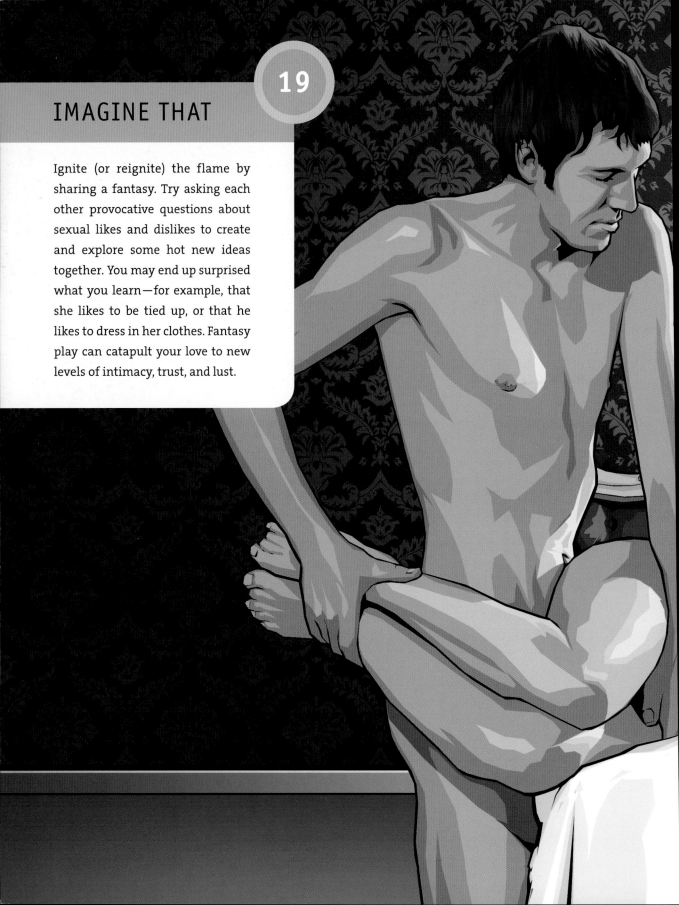

IMAGINE THAT

Ignite (or reignite) the flame by sharing a fantasy. Try asking each other provocative questions about sexual likes and dislikes to create and explore some hot new ideas together. You may end up surprised what you learn—for example, that she likes to be tied up, or that he likes to dress in her clothes. Fantasy play can catapult your love to new levels of intimacy, trust, and lust.

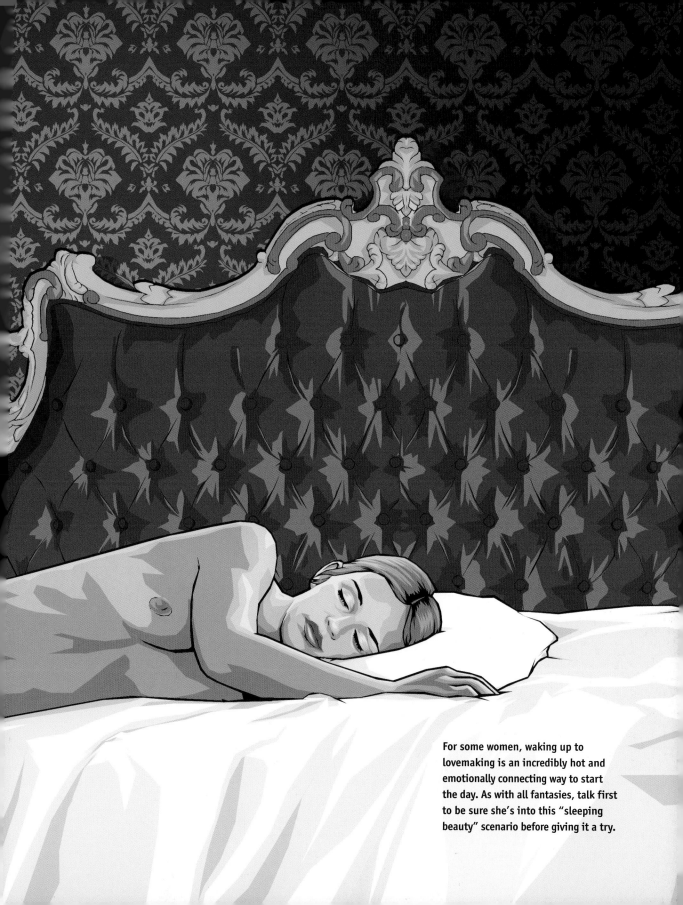

For some women, waking up to lovemaking is an incredibly hot and emotionally connecting way to start the day. As with all fantasies, talk first to be sure she's into this "sleeping beauty" scenario before giving it a try.

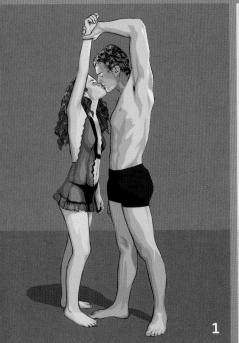

1

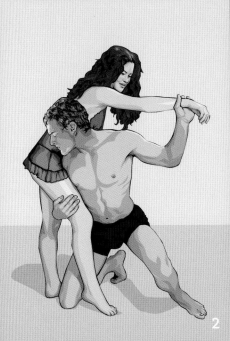

2

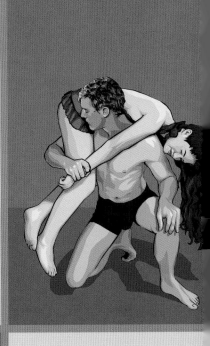

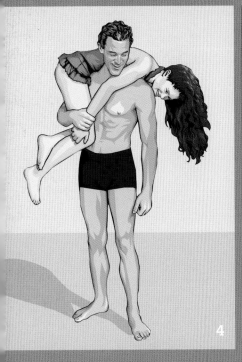

4

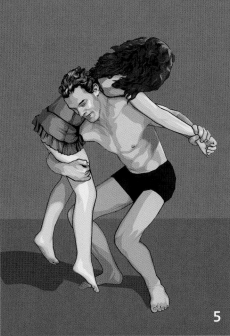

5

{1} Borrow a trick from sexy firemen and carry your lover away . . . literally. Rescuer fantasies can be flaming hot!

{2} Kneel down to protect your knees and back; with your arm between her legs, grasp one thigh firmly.

{3} Pull her over your shoulder. Grip her arm to steady her and add to the protector-and-protected feeling.

{4} Stand carefully, being sure to lift with your knees and not your back. Now you're ready to whisk her away and ravish your darling damsel.

{5} To let her down lightly, lean forward, duck your head, and roll her over your shoulder. You can gently lay her on the bed for further ravishing.

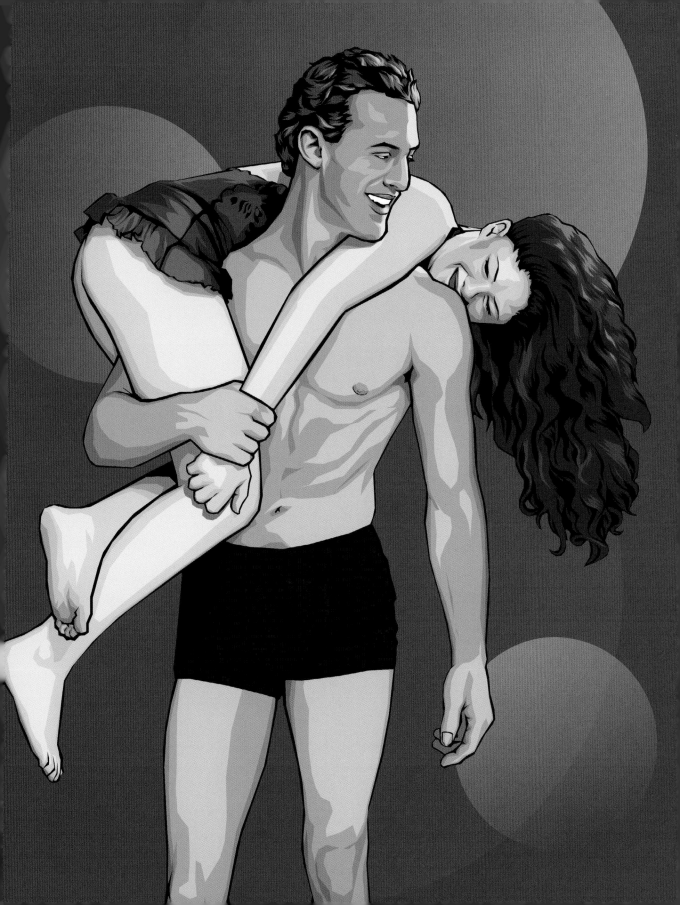

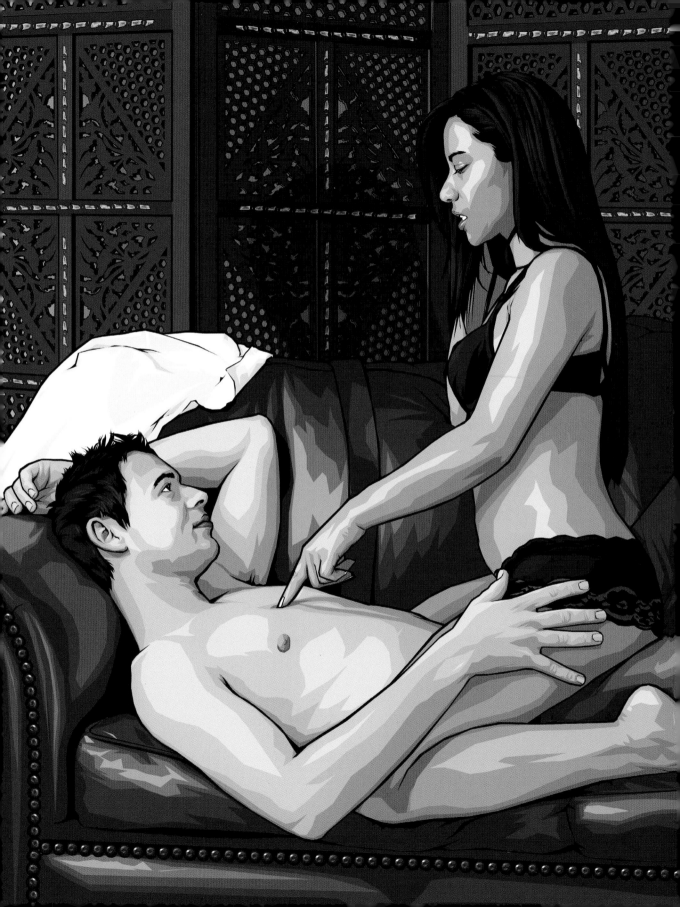

Being told what to do (or telling someone exactly how you like it done) is a steamy way to learn your lover's fantasies—and maybe discover some of your own.

DO YOU WANT TO MAKE ME? 21

Power games are a spicy way to play with your minds as well as your bodies. Many people fantasize about being dominated or about dominating a partner. Not sure? Try being, or bossing around, a sex slave for an hour (or even a few minutes) to see how it fits your personality. Then switch up your roles.

Ordering your partner to pleasure you exactly how you want—with explicit instructions—is a great tool for discovery. As you play, you may discover that you and your partner have complementary preferences: for instance, you like to be the demanding executive, while he enjoys playing the submissive secretary. If you both prefer dominating or being dominated, take turns. The key is to play nicely—even when you're getting nasty.

Want to take it a little further into dominance games? Try a spanking if your slave doesn't follow directions. Or blindfold and handcuff your slave to the chair while you feed him dinner. And after that, lead him upstairs, tie him to the bed, and show him who's boss.

Many women find oral sex to be most pleasurable when they're on their backs. Why not find out if that's true for you by experimenting with different positions?

22 CUNNILINGUS BASICS

Comfort is queen in many oral positions. Sit her on a chair, couch, or bed and spread her legs wide enough for you to enjoy the view and the experience.

Tease the inside of her thighs and her labia before you head to the clitoris. Use both the tip and the flat of your tongue to flick and lick. Slide your tongue in and out of her vagina, too, and remember that there's no need to go deep inside to make a powerful impression. Amplify her arousal by grabbing hold of her hips and rear to reinforce the moves you're making with your mouth. Have her pull your hair or moan when she especially approves of something you're doing.

Women tend to enjoy circular motions the most, as compared to what you often see in adult movies, where the man uses only the tip of his tongue. Instead, when you want to go for the climax, get in there and massage her clitoris and the areas all around it with your whole tongue. Pay attention to her responses and let her sighs and moans show you the way to bring her to orgasm.

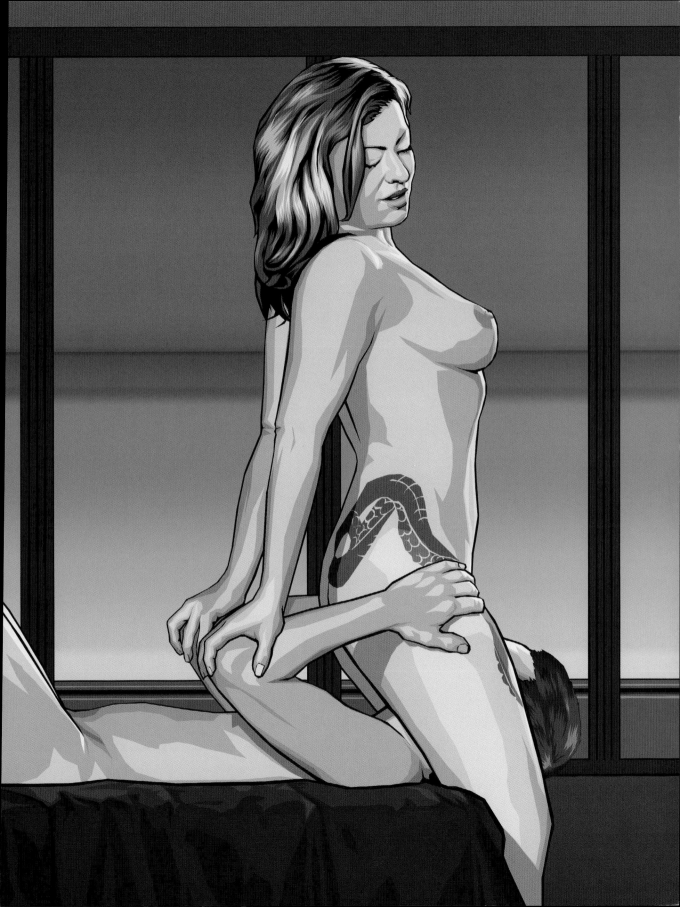

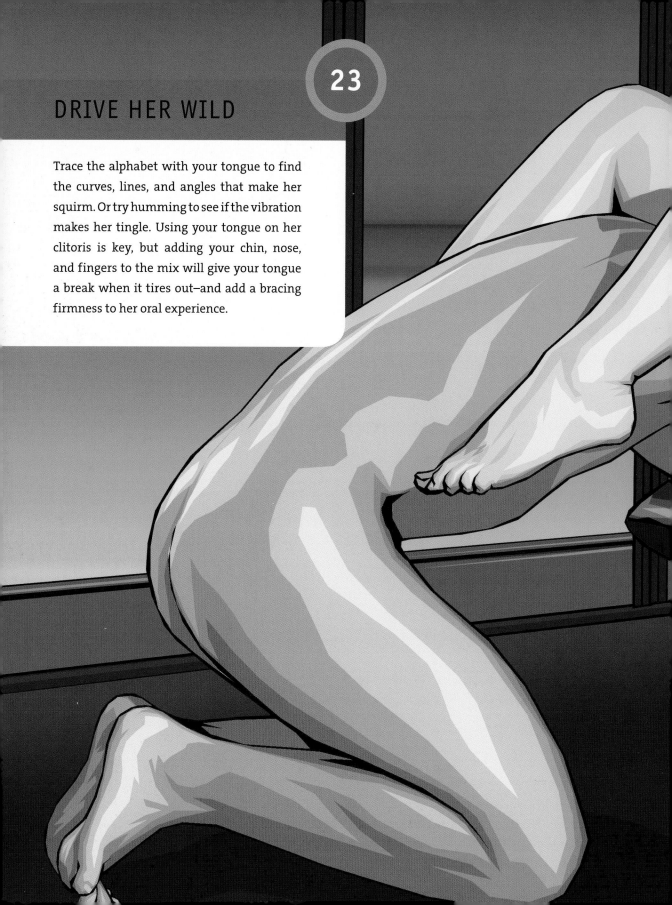

DRIVE HER WILD

Trace the alphabet with your tongue to find the curves, lines, and angles that make her squirm. Or try humming to see if the vibration makes her tingle. Using your tongue on her clitoris is key, but adding your chin, nose, and fingers to the mix will give your tongue a break when it tires out–and add a bracing firmness to her oral experience.

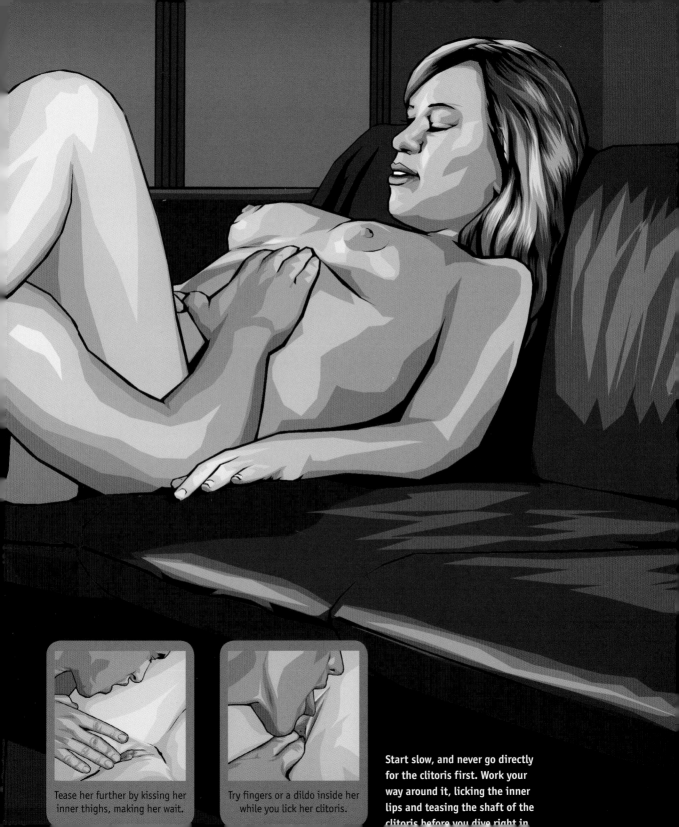

Tease her further by kissing her inner thighs, making her wait.

Try fingers or a dildo inside her while you lick her clitoris.

Start slow, and never go directly for the clitoris first. Work your way around it, licking the inner lips and teasing the shaft of the clitoris before you dive right in

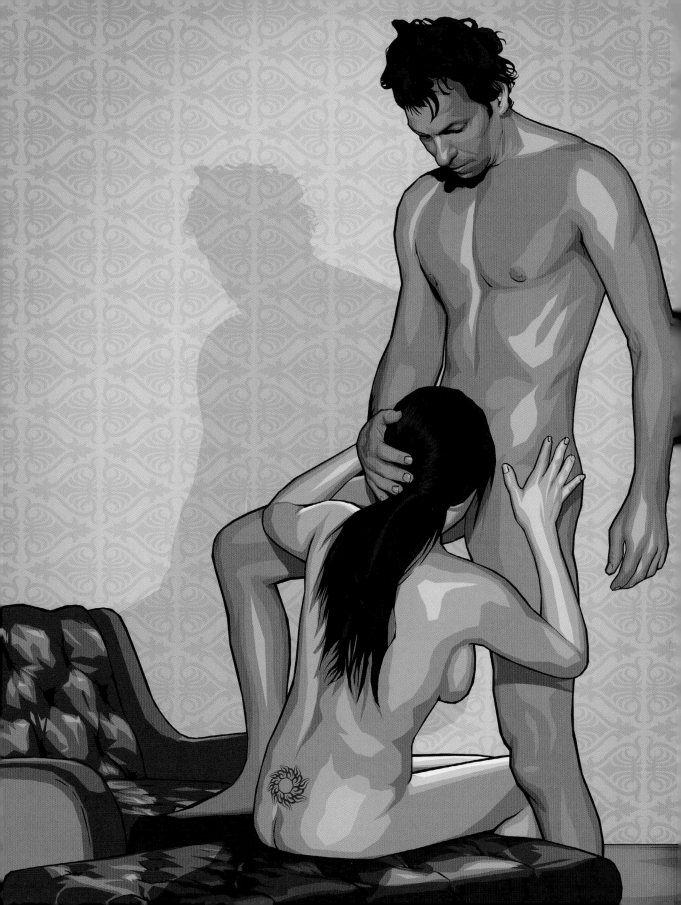

When it comes to oral sex, the real secret isn't some cryptic technique, but simple enthusiasm. If you show him how much you're enjoying yourself, he'll be thrilled.

FANTASTIC FELLATIO 24

It may be nicknamed a blow job, but it's not about blowing. And it's not strictly about moving your mouth up and down his penis, either. It's more about using your hands, mouth, tongue, and teeth (sometimes—and gently) for a range of sensations that will bring him to ecstasy.

Start before his penis even gets hard. Hold it in your hand while you kiss his inner thighs just below his testicles. Lick around the head of the penis. When you want to take more of him in, sit or stand up, whichever leaves your mouth and throat best aligned with the curve of his penis. Often, the woman-on-top position is optimal not just for 69 (a position in which partners engage in simultaneous oral sex), but for fellatio, too.

And remember, this sex act is not just oral, it's aural. Most men like noise, so let him hear your enjoyment through muffled moans. Take a break for breath (while continuing to stroke him with your hands), smile sweetly, and tell him that you like it. Then show him how sexy it makes you feel to give him pleasure.

TRICKS OF THE TONGUE

Before you go all out moving up and down, lick your way up his shaft, ending with a circling motion around the head. If he's uncircumcised, tease his foreskin. Press his testicles against his shaft, or gently tug them down. When he's really aroused, slide your fingers back and gently press the perineum (the area between his scrotum and anus).

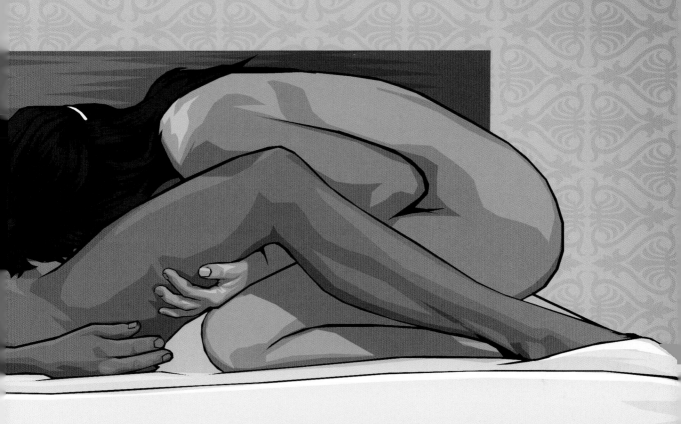

Get to know—and love—the frenulum. That's the "V" shape on the underside of his penis where the head meets the shaft. For most men, it's the single most sensitive spot. Make out with it.

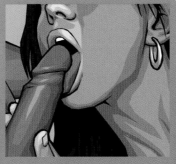

Tap the head of his penis on the tip of your tongue for a hot visual.

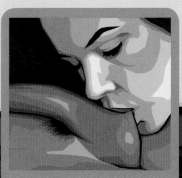

Gently lavish attention on his testicles with your mouth and hands.

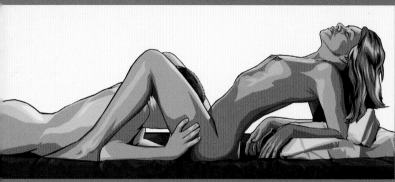

1 To maximize clitoral stimulation, women can thrust the pelvis forward, directly or by arching the back.

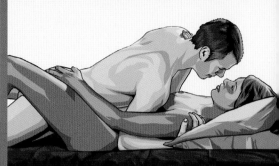

2 The tastiest lovemaking has a range of flavors. Try going from oral sex to intercourse, then back to oral.

On many people's personal list of pleasures, oral sex is an all-time favorite. But even the best things in life can be enhanced by a little variety. The key to keeping things exciting is to mix it up. It's common to get things started with the hands, move on to oral sex, and then have intercourse. But the acts we often treat as appetizers can also be delicious as the main event. So throw out the hierarchies by changing your usual order of sex acts; the types of sex you have (manual, oral, vaginal, anal); and the positions you try. Consider starting with intercourse and ending with a lavish make-out session.

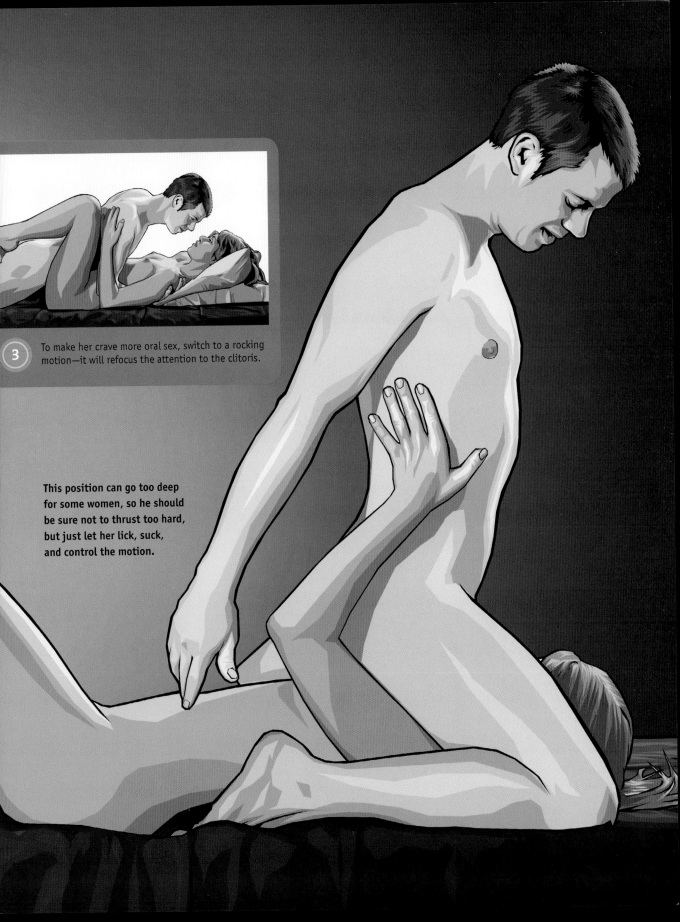

3 To make her crave more oral sex, switch to a rocking motion—it will refocus the attention to the clitoris.

This position can go too deep for some women, so he should be sure not to thrust too hard, but just let her lick, suck, and control the motion.

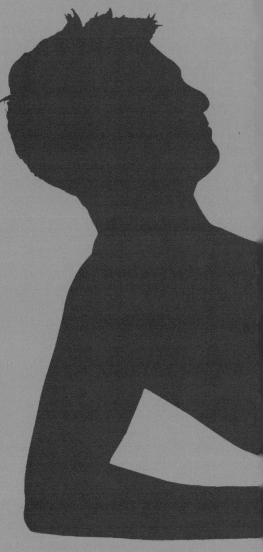

Emily

"**Why is it hot** to step into another role for a while? Because with your new identity you're more likely to diminish your inhibitions and be more primed to let loose. Role playing also enhances intimacy and puts some fun and adventure back into sex."

Jamye

"**Whether you're** dressing up in costumes or just assuming other identities, a wig not only helps you take on some secret agent identity, but it really makes you feel like you're someone else."

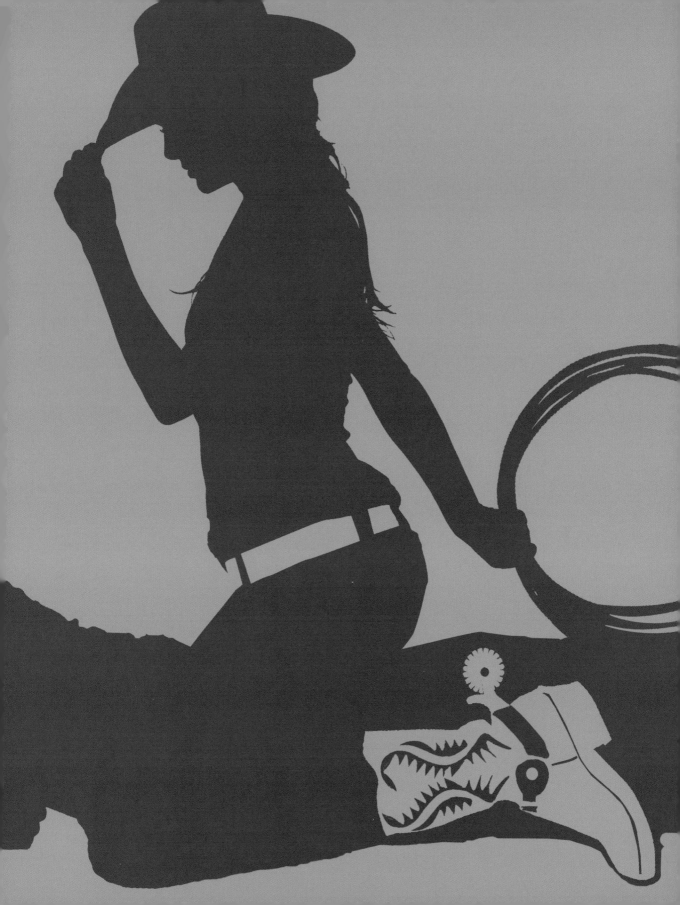

DRESS-UP FOR GROWN-UPS

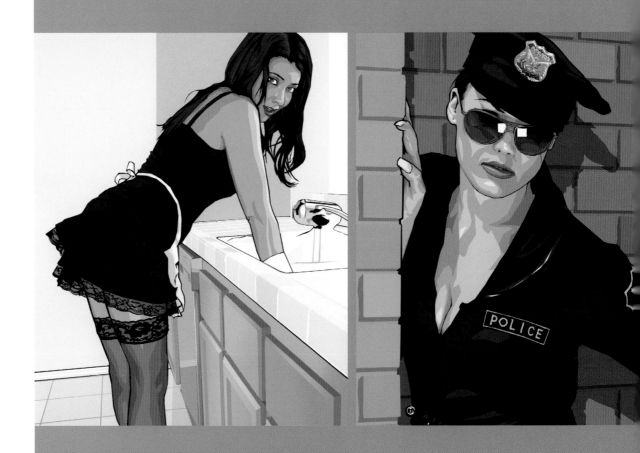

FRENCH MAID A naughty game of dress-up won't require loads of props, although a duster, apron, and sexy accent are nice additions. When you're the French maid, focus on service. Miss a spot as you scrub, and there may be sexy repercussions!

POLICEWOMAN Just who doesn't love a woman in uniform? Good cop or bad, there's a lot of power in playing a police officer, so check in with your dominant side. Even if you played the French maid yesterday, you can be a tough cop today.

COSTUMES LET YOU EXPLORE WHAT IT'S LIKE TO BE—OR DO—SOMEBODY ELSE.

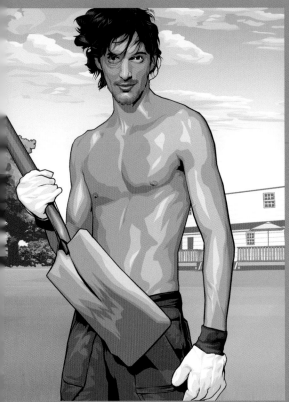 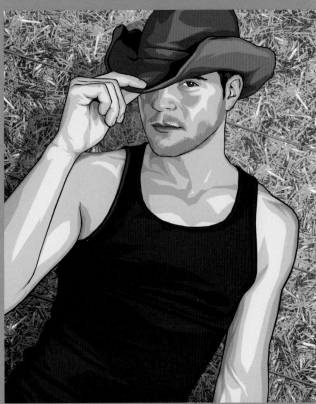

GARDENER OR POOL BOY A man who works with his hands is always welcome. For this one, you'll need to take off your shirt and be willing to work up a sweat to accommodate your employer's need for some unusually personal service.

COWBOY Swagger with style and give yourself permission to get a little rough and rugged. Cowboy hats, boots, a pair of tight jeans, and a flashy belt buckle will help you look the part. Better yet, get creative with a lasso.

Some enchanted evening, you may meet a stranger. Or, at least, pretend to. Play this game by arriving at a bar separately and acting out a steamy seduction scene.

28 COME HERE OFTEN?

The fact that this seduction plays out in public makes it sizzle. Go to an intimate location, wearing something you know your partner can't resist. Flirt with your eyes first. If you know your partner is watching you and is okay with it, flirt with a stranger or two. Maintain eye contact with your love while talking to other men or women.

When you do "meet," use fake names. Make small talk. Brush up against each other. Buy each other a drink. Get into the roles that appeal to you, whether you're playing a couple of traveling salespeople on the prowl or a CEO who has hired a male escort to give her an evening of much-needed stress relief.

And don't leave the bar until foreplay has begun. That means light touches on the back, legs, and neck, or anywhere that's likely to generate a little electricity. Then invite that sexy "stranger" home for some torrid lovemaking. Or, complete the fantasy by whisking your partner away to a lush hotel room—or a seedy motel, depending on your fantasy.

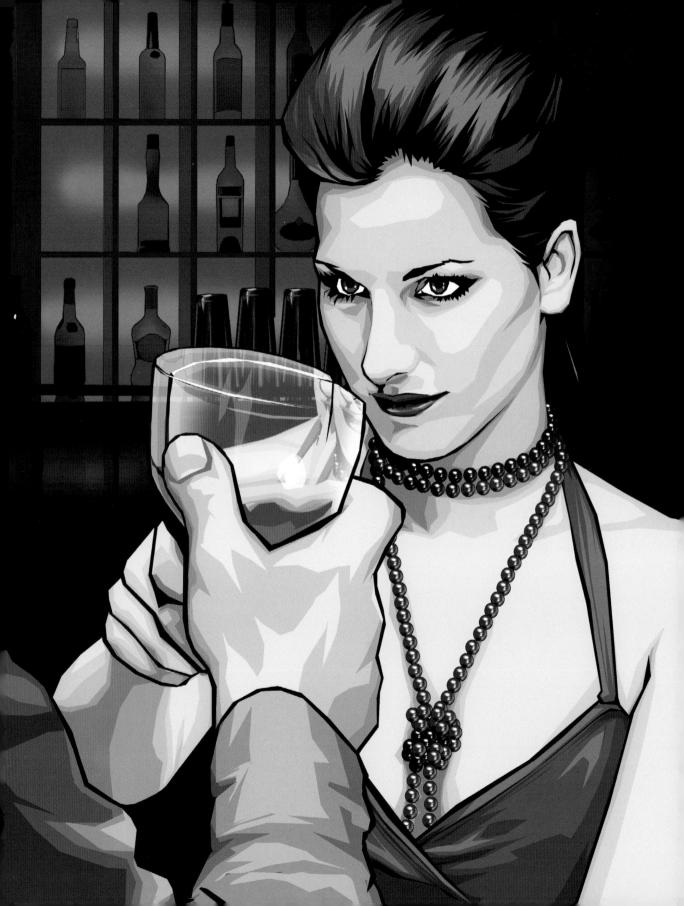

THROW DOWN

Whether you're the partner doing the hair-pulling or the one being held down, play wrestling can be silly or sexy–or a bit of both. Faux fighting gets your heart racing and your endorphins going until you're happy, sweaty, and very turned on. Try tickling some of the places that make your partner wiggle. But be sure to play fair, and stop if he or she truly objects. Tease, don't taunt!

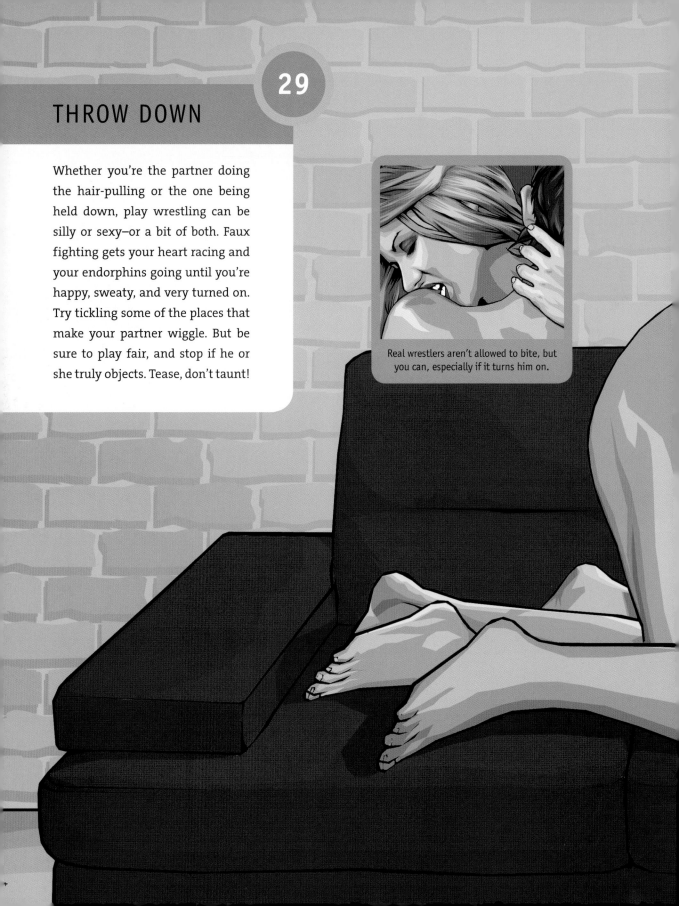

Real wrestlers aren't allowed to bite, but you can, especially if it turns him on.

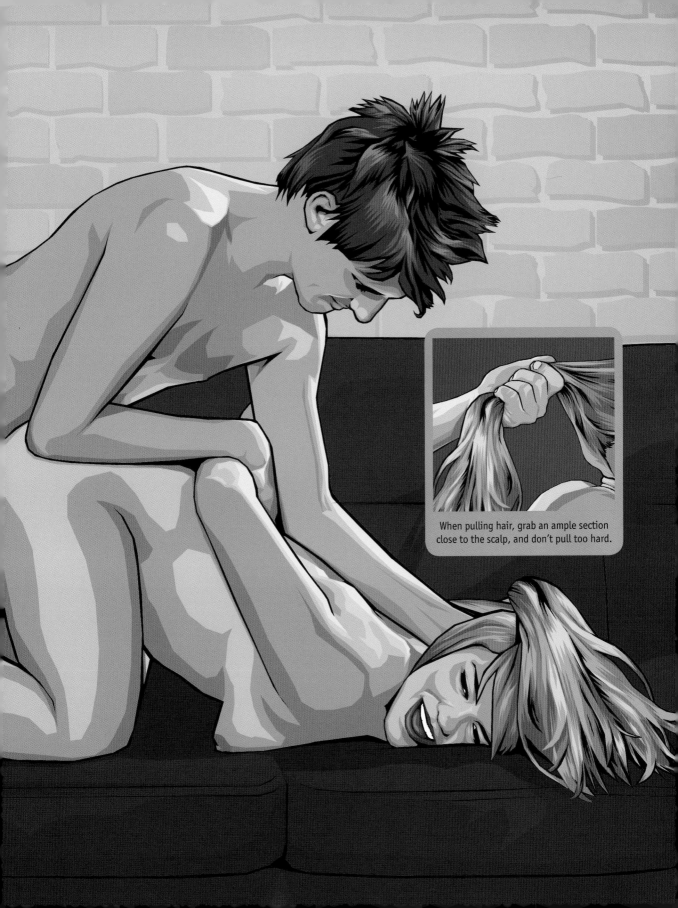

When pulling hair, grab an ample section close to the scalp, and don't pull too hard.

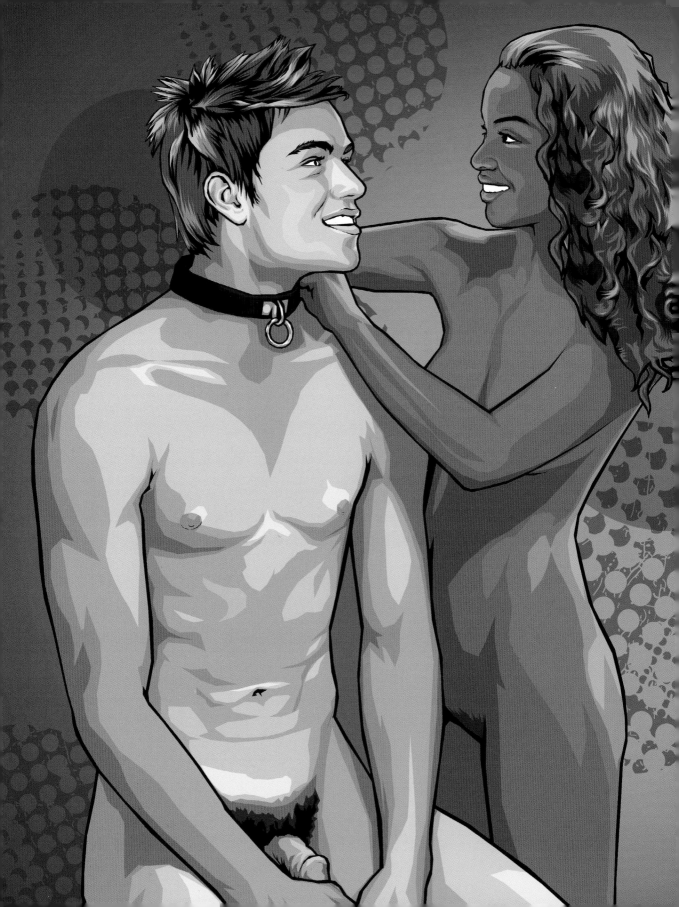

Not only does a collar look hot as a naughty accessory, but you can also grab a leash, hook it to the collar, and take your human playmate for a walk.

WHO'S A GOOD DOGGIE? 30

Even if you're pretty positive that you prefer vanilla sex, you can't be entirely sure until you've tasted other flavors. For many, BDSM (the acronym that covers bondage and discipline, dominance and submission, and sadism and masochism) satisfies exotic tastes.

Many of us really enjoy power games, whether that means whips and collars or gentle suggestion. Remember, the brain is the largest sex organ. As hot and sexy as they may be, our bodies are only as seductive as our minds let them be.

Discuss your fantasies and expectations before you begin, since role playing can unleash strong emotions. Discuss what each of you enjoys, thinks you might like, and is definitely not interested in exploring. Agree on a safe word—a term that can be used to end the session. It's especially helpful for people who enjoy pretending to resist (so you know whether to take "No, not that!" as "I'm playing" or "Stop it!"). Many couples use a system wherein "yellow" conveys "this is getting a little intense" and "red" means "stop."

31

AT THE FOOT OF IT ALL

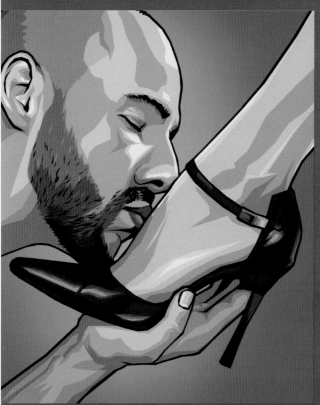

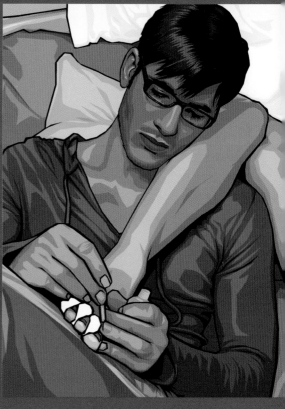

SHOE WORSHIP Whether she favors sexy stilettos or flip-flops, shoes can be sensual for both of you. If she's wearing boots, start by kissing the toes and work your way up to the laces. Bonus points if you can untie them with your teeth.

DIY PEDI Bring essentials like a nail file, pumice stone, and polish, and get into servicing your partner's feet. And don't forget to give a delicious foot massage. If you take off your clothes, you may get an especially generous tip.

HAVE FUN WITH THOSE FEET—CLAD IN SHOES, BOOTS, OR NOTHING AT ALL!

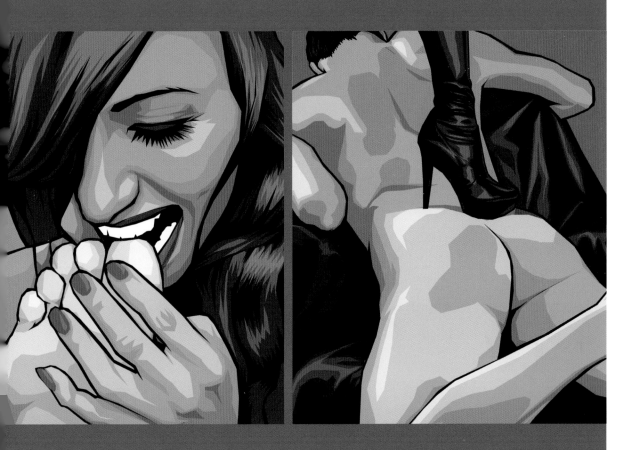

TOE JOB Nibbling and sucking on toes can be a lively part of foreplay. Pretend each one is his penis, and give all ten individual piggies a toe job. Lick up, down, and in between his toes. Finish gently by kissing the pads of each toe.

THE HIGH-HEEL HOVER If you want to try "massaging" his back with a high heel, posture is key. Stand up straight to avoid putting too much weight on him. Step heel-first and tread lightly, placing your weight only on muscular areas.

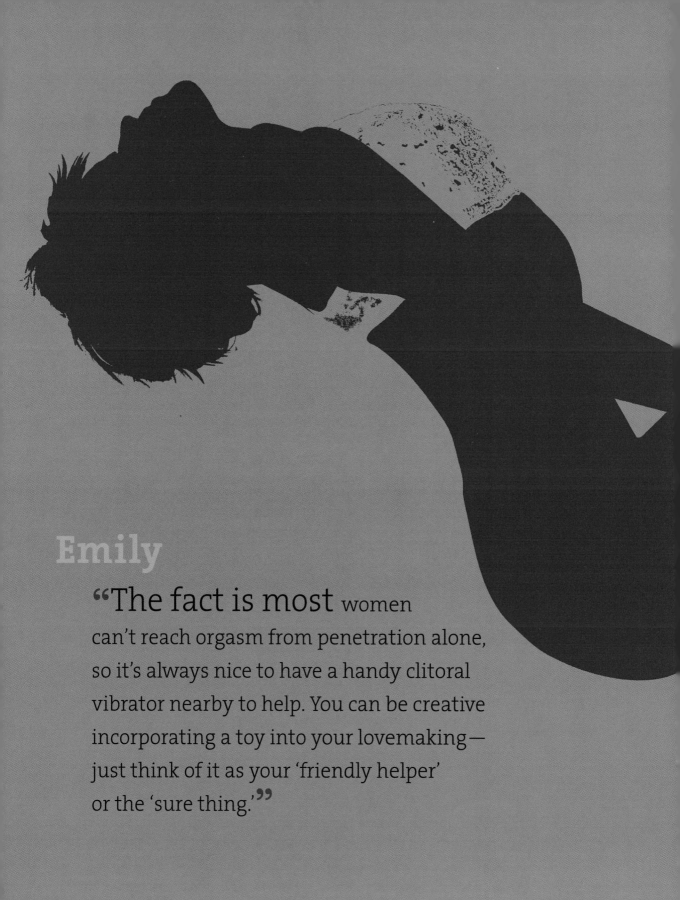

Emily

"The fact is most women can't reach orgasm from penetration alone, so it's always nice to have a handy clitoral vibrator nearby to help. You can be creative incorporating a toy into your lovemaking—just think of it as your 'friendly helper' or the 'sure thing.'"

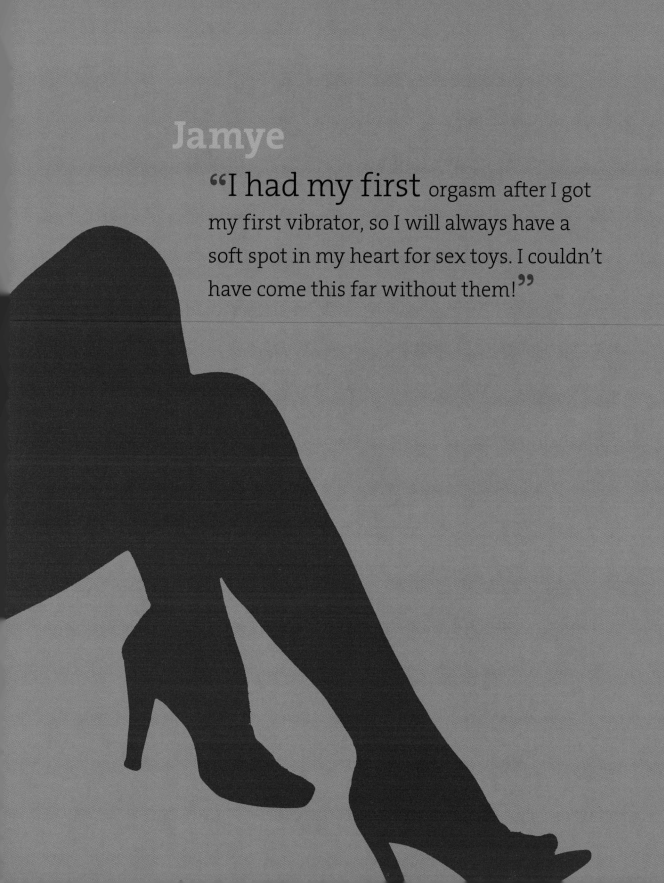

Jamye

"I had my first orgasm after I got my first vibrator, so I will always have a soft spot in my heart for sex toys. I couldn't have come this far without them!"

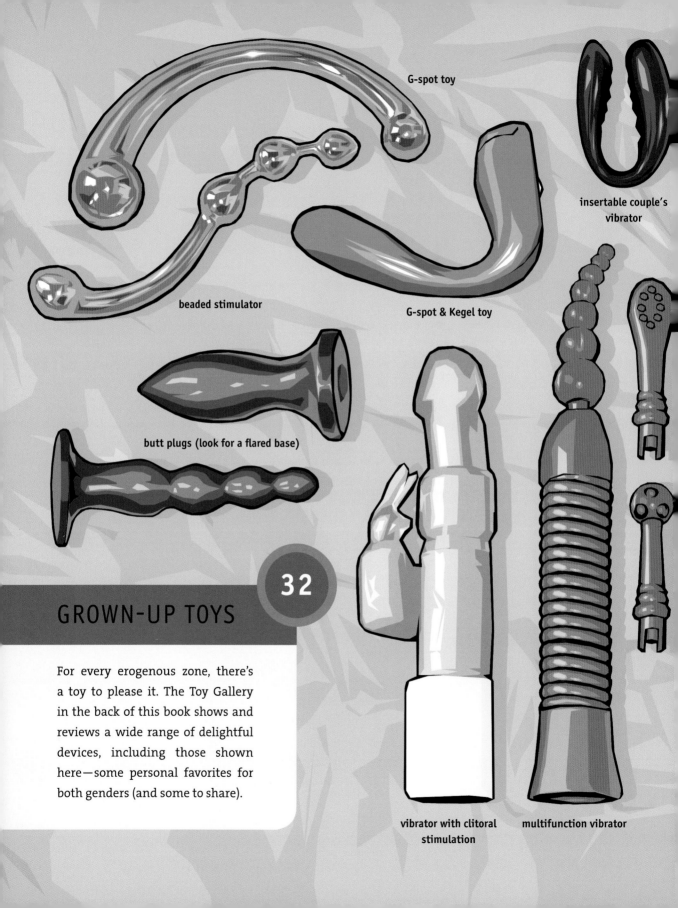

G-spot toy

insertable couple's vibrator

beaded stimulator

G-spot & Kegel toy

butt plugs (look for a flared base)

32

GROWN-UP TOYS

For every erogenous zone, there's a toy to please it. The Toy Gallery in the back of this book shows and reviews a wide range of delightful devices, including those shown here—some personal favorites for both genders (and some to share).

vibrator with clitoral stimulation

multifunction vibrator

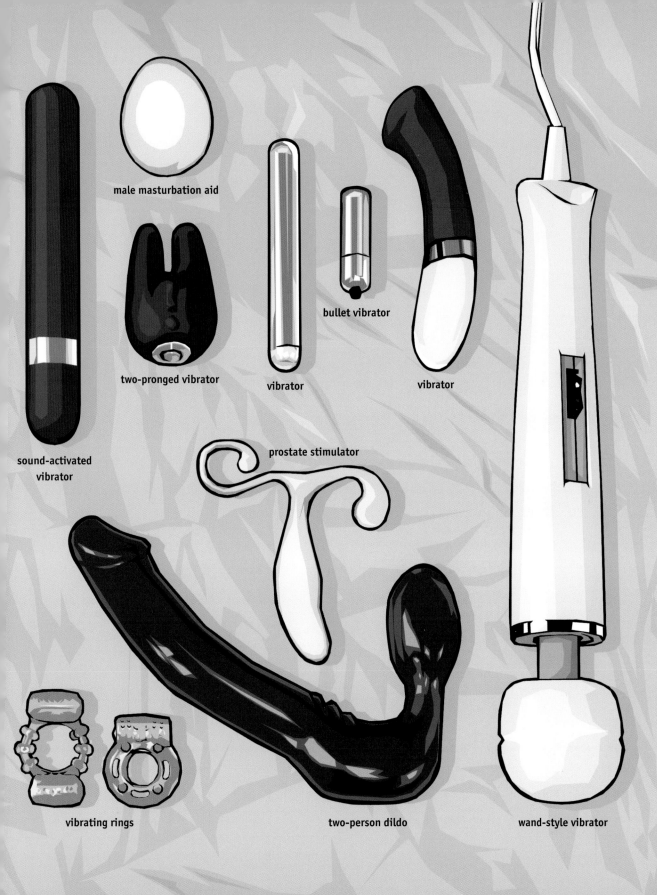

male masturbation aid

two-pronged vibrator

vibrator

bullet vibrator

vibrator

sound-activated
vibrator

prostate stimulator

vibrating rings

two-person dildo

wand-style vibrator

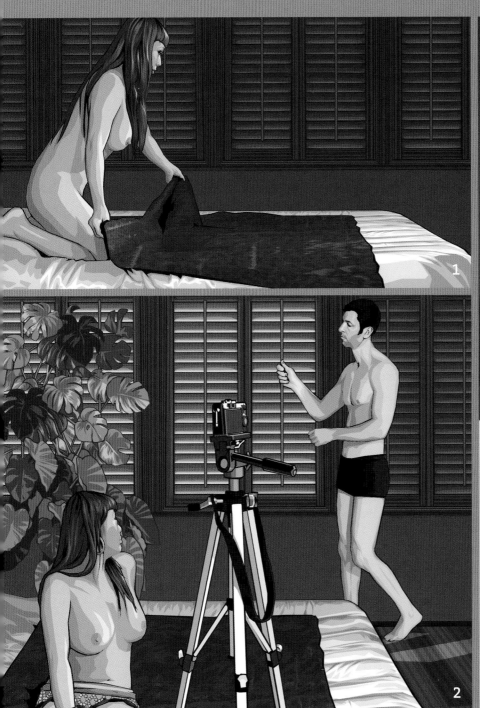

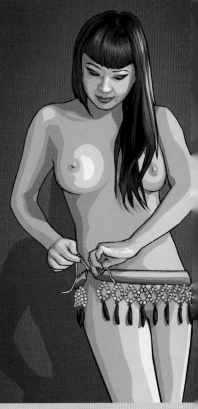

{1} Set the stage. Be sure your environment is inviting. Clear away distractions like lamps or clutter.

{2} Close the blinds for privacy, and use diffused natural light, which is the most flattering. Multiple lamps work better than a spotlight.

{3} Just a few little costume pieces can create a character—anything from jungle princess to saucy schoolgirl.

{4} Shoot straight on to maximize assets, or from above to minimize. Relax and enjoy the attention and your sexy connection.

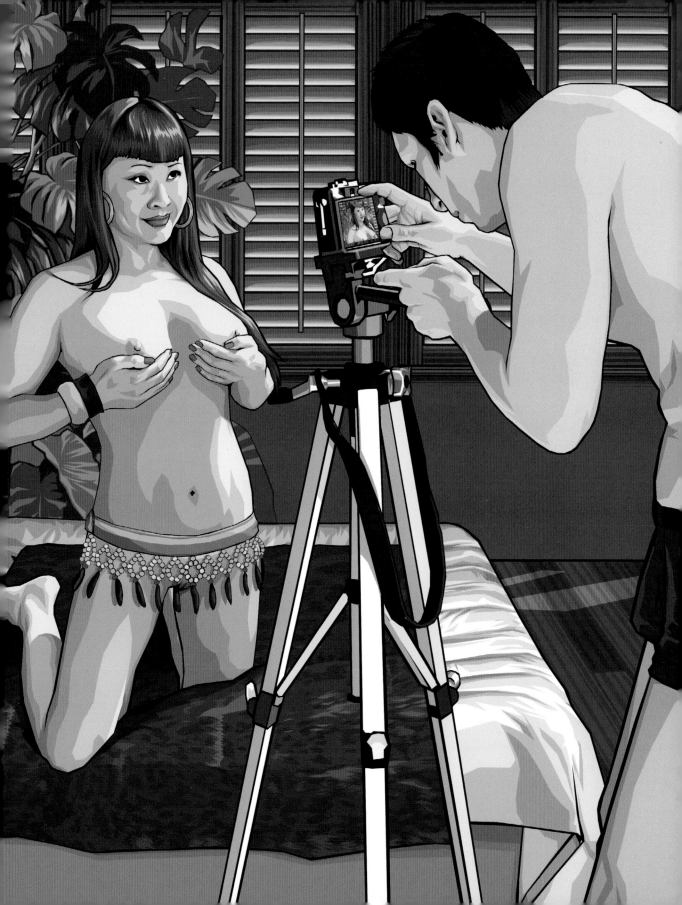

ENTWINE

There are really only six basic sex positions. It's true—all of the amazing and delightful things two bodies can do together are simply creative variations on one of the following: missionary, woman on top, spooning, doggie, sitting, or standing. Most people have a couple of favorites— those two or three things you know always work to get you excited, build connection, or get you there. But there are so many possibilities for mixing it up. Sometimes it's as easy as wrapping a leg or moving your hands in a different way—small changes that make a spine-tingling difference. Sometimes, it's all about location. You can make your home into your own sexy gymnasium, and try out new things in the bedroom or the shower, on the stairs, or all over your sofa. Remember, you don't have to do positions in any set order. You can combine the positions in this book in new ways, or create your own. Flip through these pages and see which ideas grab you—and then grab your partner and go with what feels right, exciting, challenging, and fun.

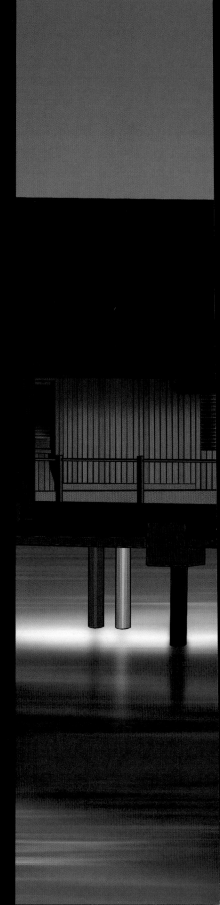

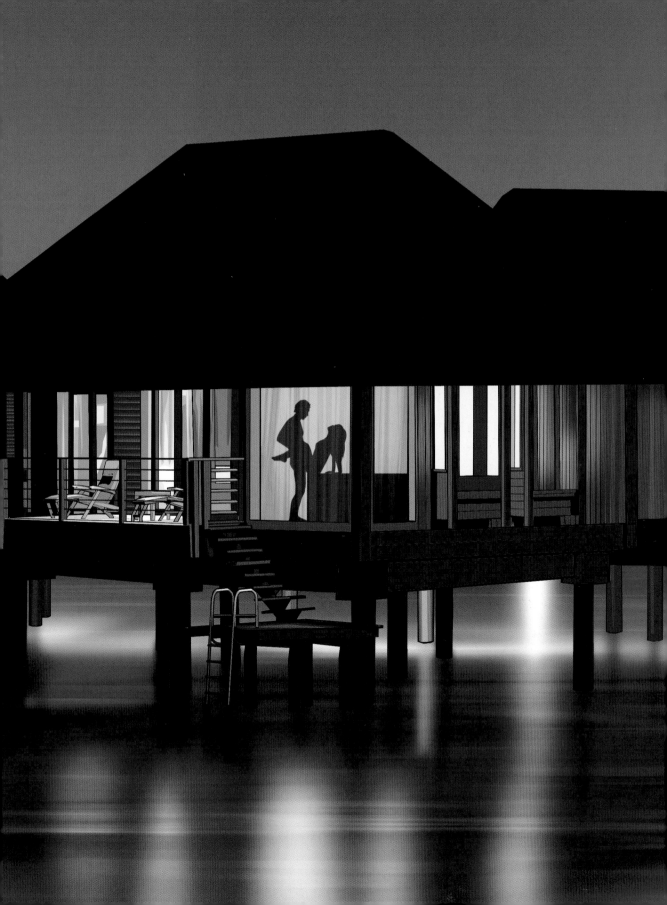

Having sex standing up conveys desire at its strongest: wanting your partner so intensely that the two of you can't even make it to the couch or bedroom.

34 TAKING A STAND

Nothing says, "I need to have you now" like doing it standing up. More than any other position, it expresses a powerful urgency, especially if you don't even take the time to get fully undressed.

Standing positions involve a unique set of challenges, including differing partner height, strength, balance, and coordination. Sound difficult? You don't have to make this a freestanding event. Lean on your lover for support or against a handy wall. In a more narrow door frame, you can both brace your arms and legs in interesting ways. Do be careful with your movements—a slip can end up bending him in ways that are just no fun.

It might take a little experimentation, but if you adjust as you go, it'll all work out. Start out with her spreading her legs, bending her knees, and facing forward or backward. He can also lift her up against the wall, with both her legs wrapped around his waist. Or she can try standing on one leg while wrapping her other leg around him. That's a classic standing position—and for good reason.

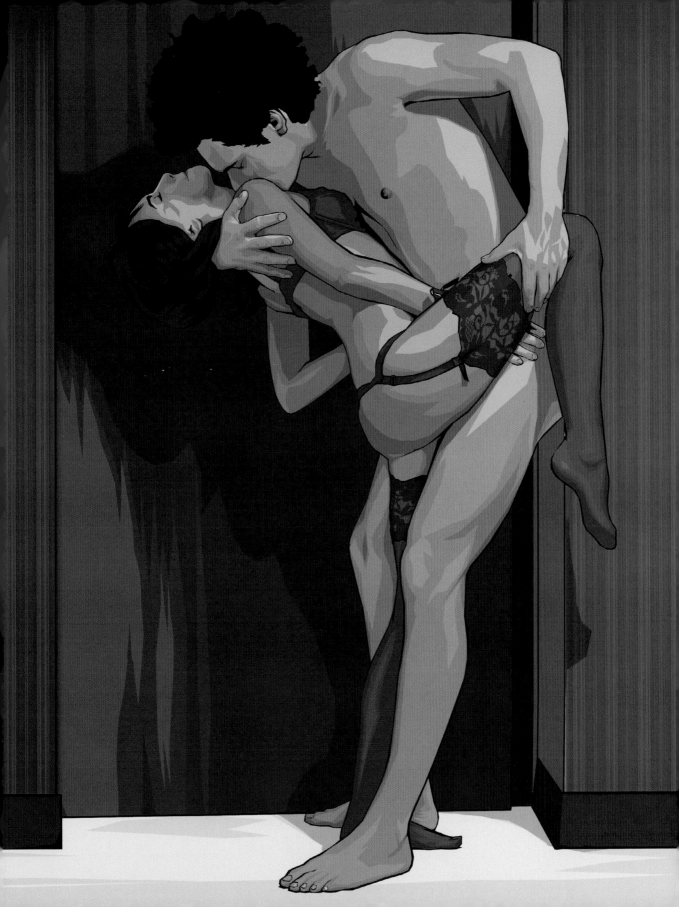

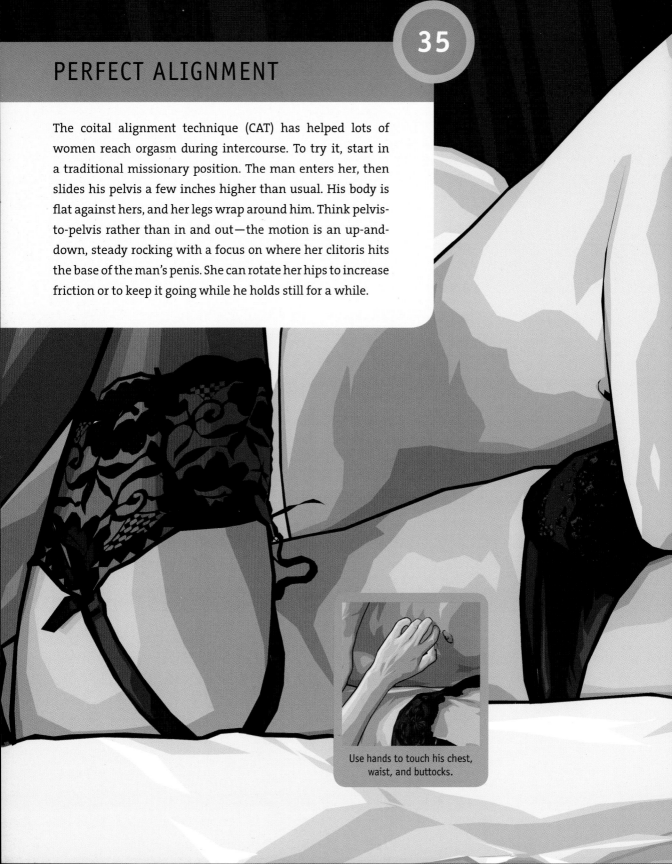

PERFECT ALIGNMENT

The coital alignment technique (CAT) has helped lots of women reach orgasm during intercourse. To try it, start in a traditional missionary position. The man enters her, then slides his pelvis a few inches higher than usual. His body is flat against hers, and her legs wrap around him. Think pelvis-to-pelvis rather than in and out—the motion is an up-and-down, steady rocking with a focus on where her clitoris hits the base of the man's penis. She can rotate her hips to increase friction or to keep it going while he holds still for a while.

Use hands to touch his chest, waist, and buttocks.

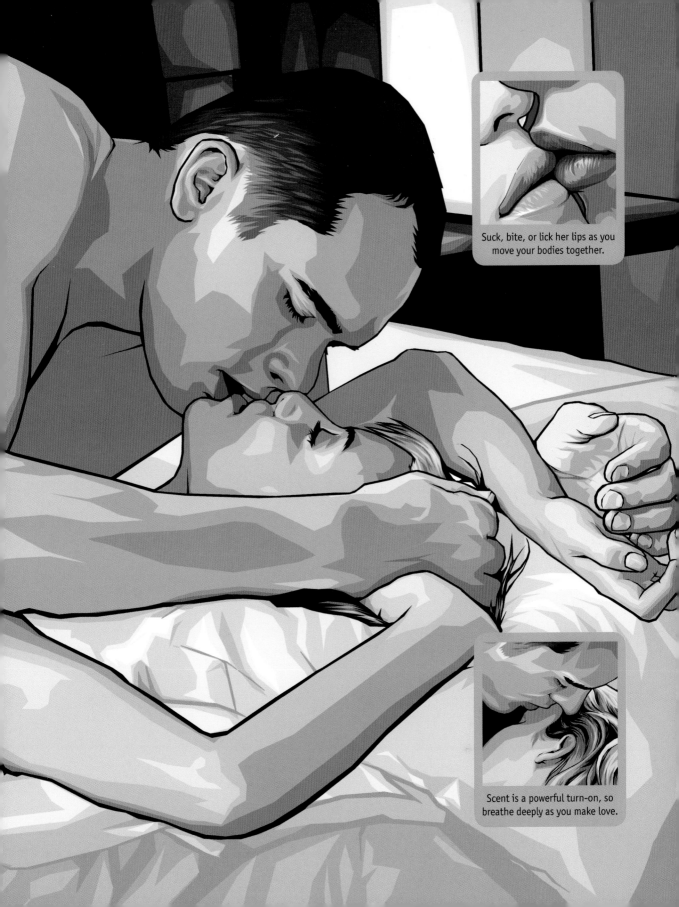

Suck, bite, or lick her lips as you move your bodies together.

Scent is a powerful turn-on, so breathe deeply as you make love.

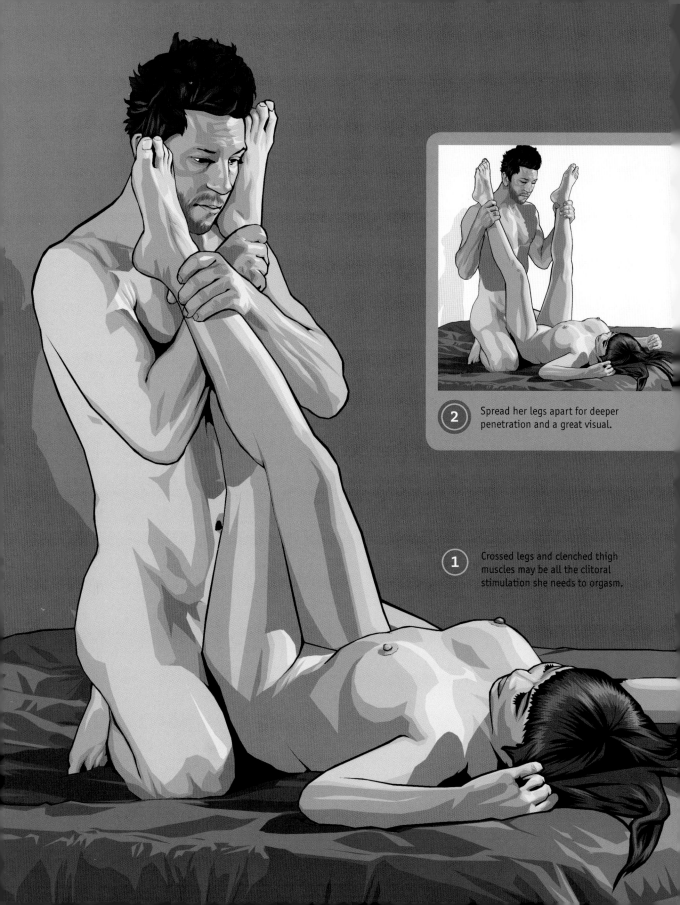

2 Spread her legs apart for deeper penetration and a great visual.

1 Crossed legs and clenched thigh muscles may be all the clitoral stimulation she needs to orgasm.

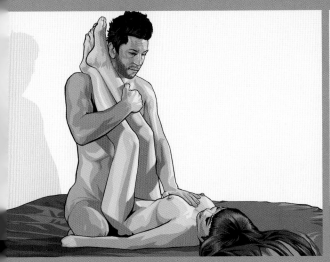

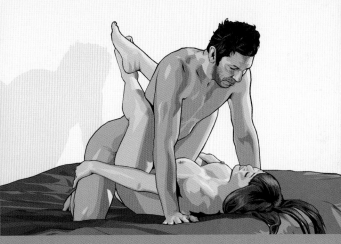

 3 Place her legs over one of your shoulders to hit new angles inside of her. Also try switching shoulders.

4 Bring her knees down around your waist for a slightly shallower thrust and a sense of connection.

The man-on-top position has a reputation for being less exciting—but that's only if it's the only way you do it every time you do it.

There are plenty of spicy variations on the missionary theme. Make it your mission to try out a few. For instance, raising a woman's legs will increase the intensity of the man's thrusts. Or she can squeeze her legs together, which keeps him from thrusting too deeply and makes everything down there feel tighter. When he holds her ankles, it adds an element of power play.

Each of these positions can feel radically different with just slight adjustments of her legs—try them higher or lower, closer together or widely spread, and propped on one or both shoulders. Most missionary variations can be great if you're having anal sex, too. If that's the case, you'll get a better angle if you place a pillow under her butt.

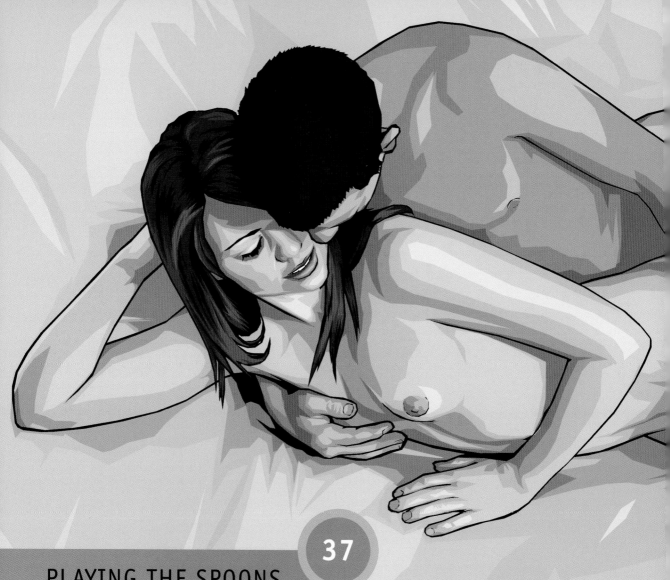

PLAYING THE SPOONS

A spooning session is as easy as waking up, rolling over, and getting it on. A man and woman just need to lie on their sides as he enters her from behind. This is a great option whether you're sleepy, pregnant, or you're just feeling cuddly. To take it up a notch, she can bend up her top knee, place her hand between her thighs, and fondle his testicles.

Spooning positions are great if she prefers shallow penetration, but you can take it deeper by transitioning to doggie-style. He can lift one of her legs and enjoy the spooning position for a while, and then, when both are ready, roll her over onto her belly or knees and continue.

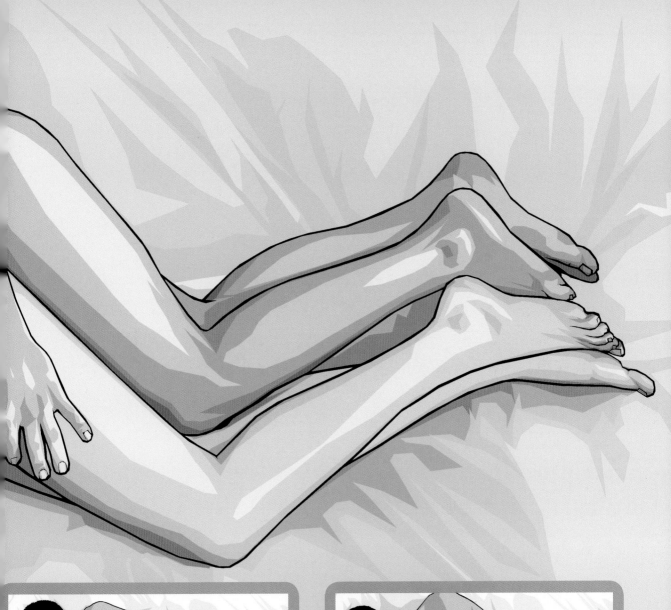

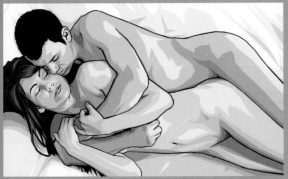

Take the opportunity to focus on your connection, since you're pressed together and the position doesn't require much energy.

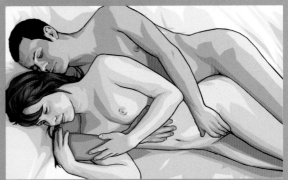

His hands are free to hold her close, stroke her breasts, belly, and hips, or play with her clitoris. She can touch herself, too.

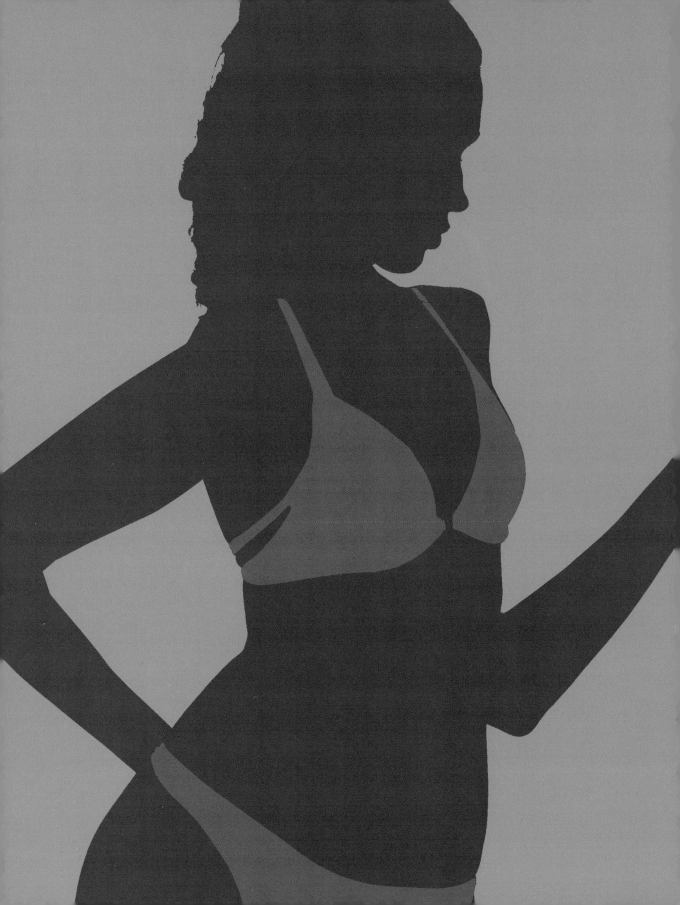

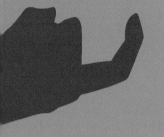

Emily

"**Woman on top** is a win-win situation. She's in control of the motion, intensity, and thrusting, and her partner gets to take in the whole picture. Men are intensely visual, and they're getting the best seat in the house with this one."

Jamye

"**I don't know much** that's sexier than a woman who knows what she wants and how to get it, and that's what makes woman-on-top positions so hot. She gets to control everything from the angle to the orgasm."

When a woman's on top, she's in charge of the action. And because the man has a limited range of motion, it may make the sexual encounter last longer. Giddyup!

38 RIDE HIM, COWGIRL

At once passionate and personal, the cowgirl position is a popular favorite. To make it work for you, straddle your partner with your knees on either side of his hips. You can also squat over his body with your feet flat on the outer sides of his thighs. Either way, the key is to slowly lower yourself, and ease him inside.

If you're both sitting up, you can press yourselves chest to chest and cheek to cheek. Intimate eye contact is almost unavoidable. While you're gazing deeply, smile and wrap your hands around your partner's body, or place them on the back of the chair, couch, or bed to use as leverage. Or lean away from him, arch your back, and give him a show.

You can ride your man all sorts of ways. Move up and down, rock back and forth, or grind your hips in a circle. Try squeezing your pelvic floor muscles, too. Some women feel self-conscious about being "on display" in this way, but trust us: your partner loves a sexy show. This position is also convenient—when she's wearing a skirt, it can happen anywhere.

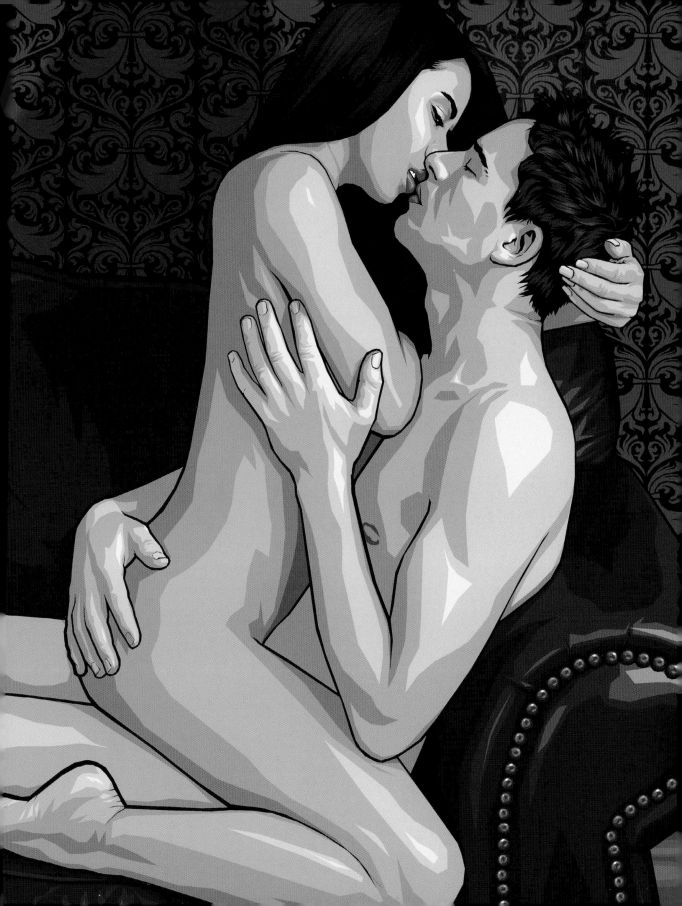

One great thing about her being on top is that she can move her pelvis to hit her G-spot and A-spot (farther up on the top wall of the vaginal canal, closer to the cervix). Plus, her clitoris is easily accessible to her own hands or those of her partner.

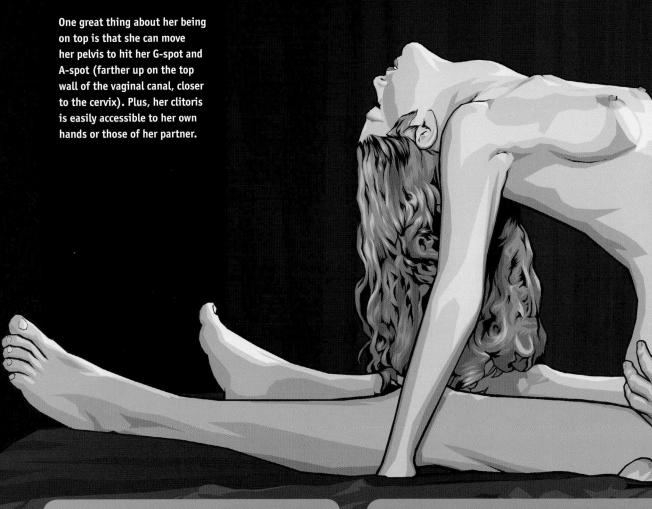

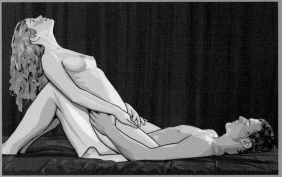

When he bends his knees, she can lean back for support. It also allows her to target the sensitive area around her G-spot.

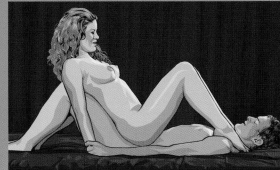

Play with leg position to vary the penetration depth. This angle allows him to go deeper. Squeezing her thighs helps, too.

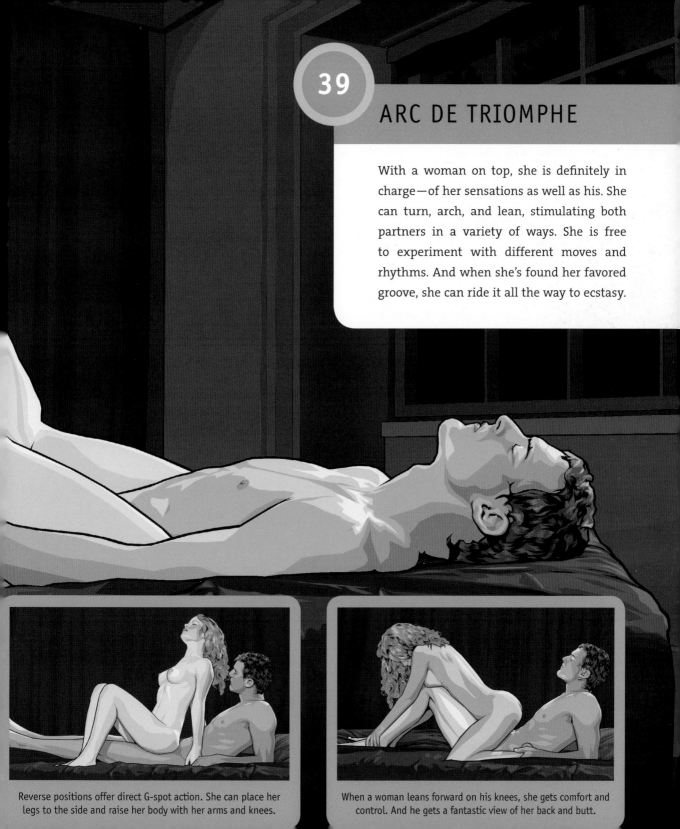

39

ARC DE TRIOMPHE

With a woman on top, she is definitely in charge—of her sensations as well as his. She can turn, arch, and lean, stimulating both partners in a variety of ways. She is free to experiment with different moves and rhythms. And when she's found her favored groove, she can ride it all the way to ecstasy.

Reverse positions offer direct G-spot action. She can place her legs to the side and raise her body with her arms and knees.

When a woman leans forward on his knees, she gets comfort and control. And he gets a fantastic view of her back and butt.

40

HIT HER HOT SPOTS

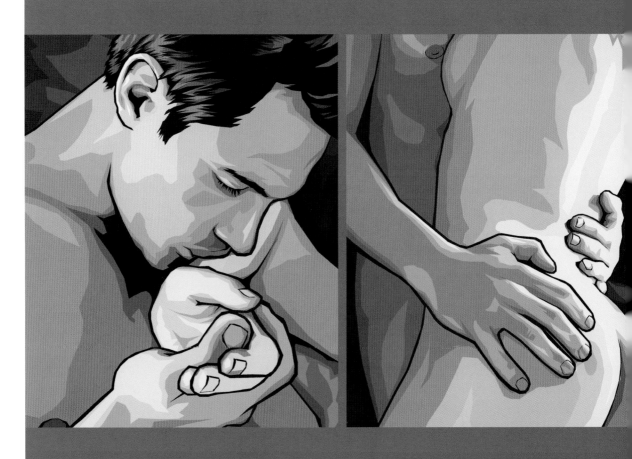

1 **ROAM THE TERRAIN** Start at the wrists. Lick them. Breathe on them. Use your tongue to make slow circles up and down from hand to elbow. Spread the love by moving slowly up and down every inch of her body.

2 **PULL HER IN CLOSE** Next time you're going in for a kiss, wrap your hands around her waist. Grab her butt. Press her body into yours. The more you touch her, the more excited she'll get— and the more she'll touch you.

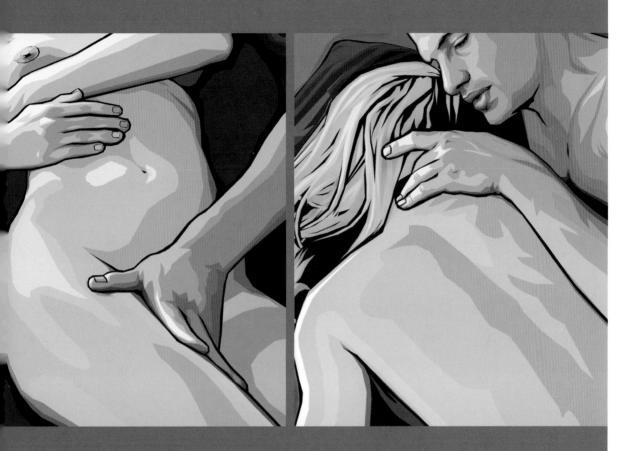

3 **BUILD EXCITEMENT** Even though clitoral stimulation is the best way for most women to reach orgasm, take your time going there. Stroke her hips and inner thighs, then move slowly toward her mound and outer lips.

4 **BREATHE EASY** The nape of the neck is one of the sexiest go-to places on most bodies. Gently massage this area to release energy and to build sexual tension. Light kisses work well, as does a bit of up-close heavy breathing.

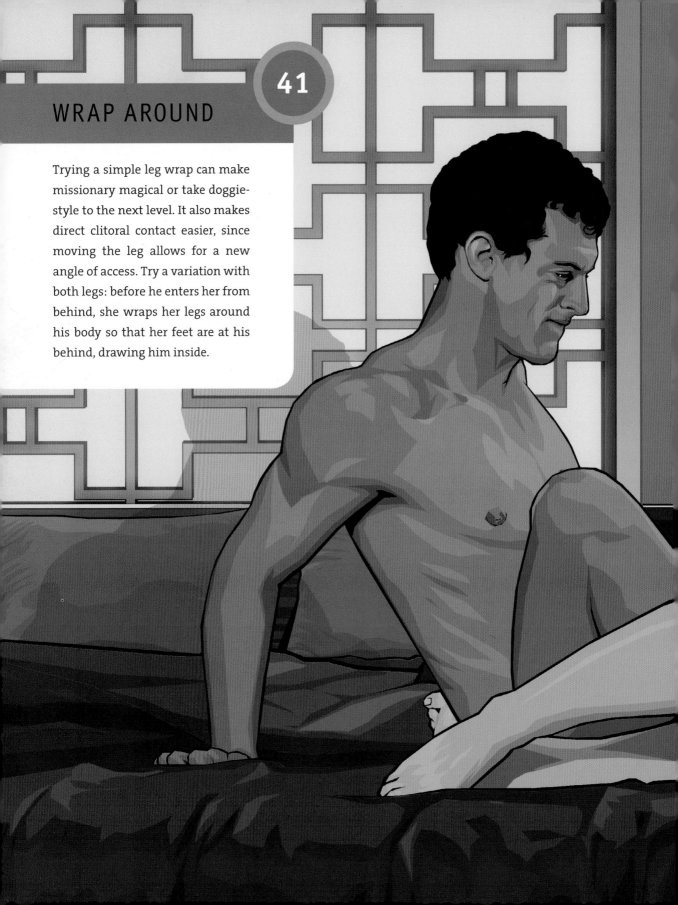

41

WRAP AROUND

Trying a simple leg wrap can make missionary magical or take doggie-style to the next level. It also makes direct clitoral contact easier, since moving the leg allows for a new angle of access. Try a variation with both legs: before he enters her from behind, she wraps her legs around his body so that her feet are at his behind, drawing him inside.

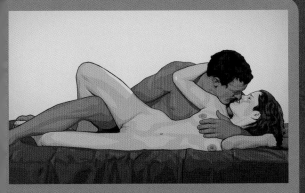

Open up your spooning style. With her leg wrapped around his thigh, there's more room for hands-on clitoral stimulation.

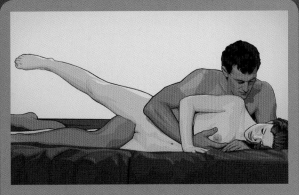

With her top leg extended straight out and his top knee bent, he can use his thigh to directly massage her clitoris.

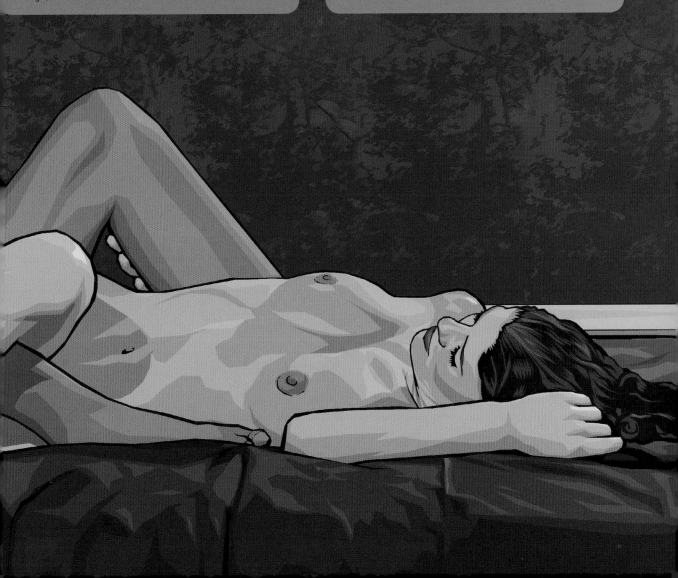

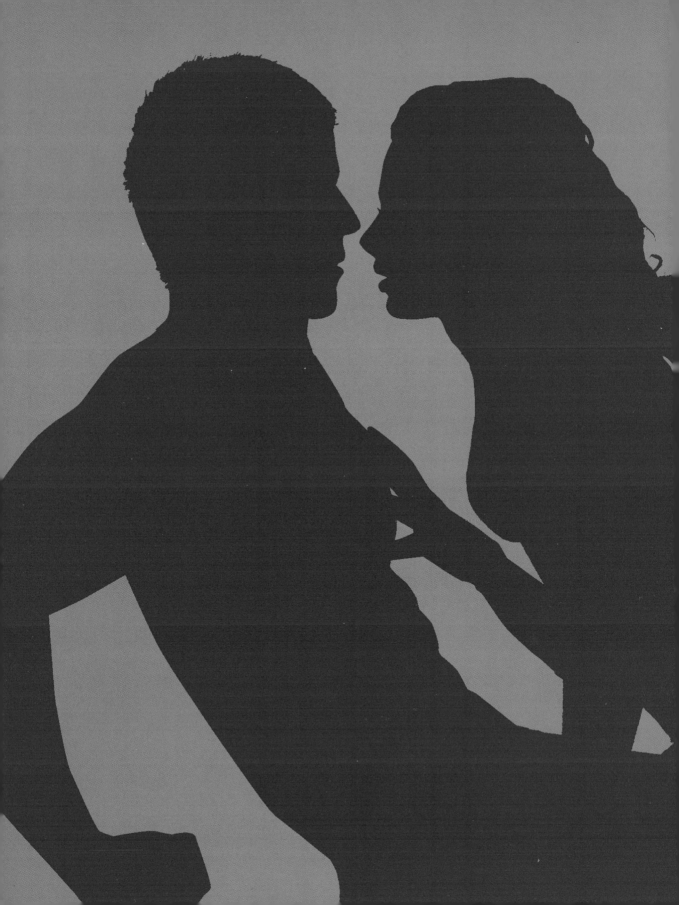

Emily

"Getting in touch with what you want and need in the moment can be a real turn-on. The next step is expressing this to your partner. If you know what you want, just ask for it. Don't worry. It gets easier with practice. Then be sure to listen to what your partner wants as well!"

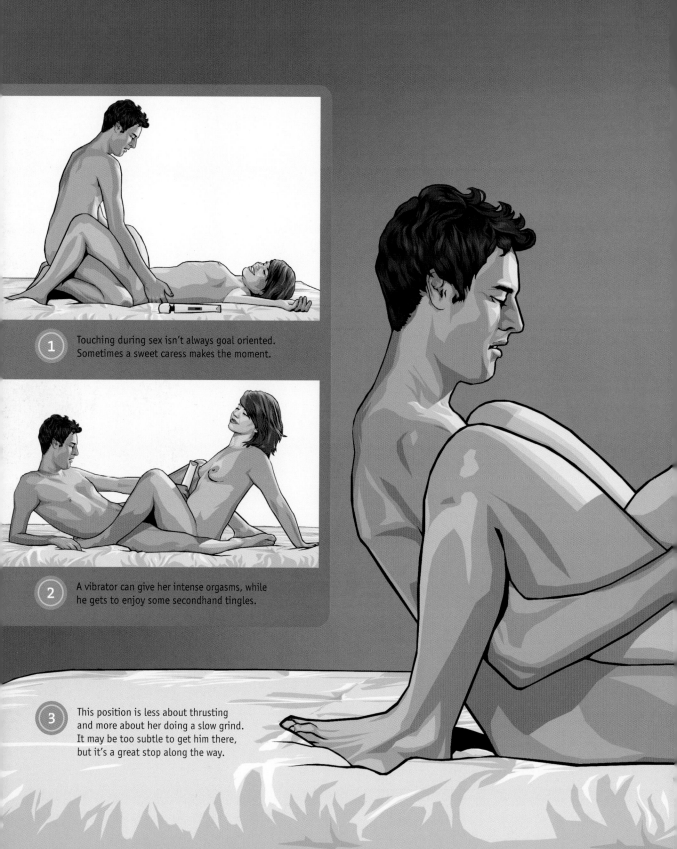

1. Touching during sex isn't always goal oriented. Sometimes a sweet caress makes the moment.

2. A vibrator can give her intense orgasms, while he gets to enjoy some secondhand tingles.

3. This position is less about thrusting and more about her doing a slow grind. It may be too subtle to get him there, but it's a great stop along the way.

While not every sex session absolutely has to end with an orgasm, it's certainly a nice bit of punctuation for the end (and the middle, and sometimes the beginning). The big bang may occur as a result of penetration, but you might want to experiment with a range of other techniques to get there. You can explore vibrators, dildos, and other sex toys—but don't forget your hands and even your feet. You can enhance your sex life and celebrate your connection with every part of your body—and then some.

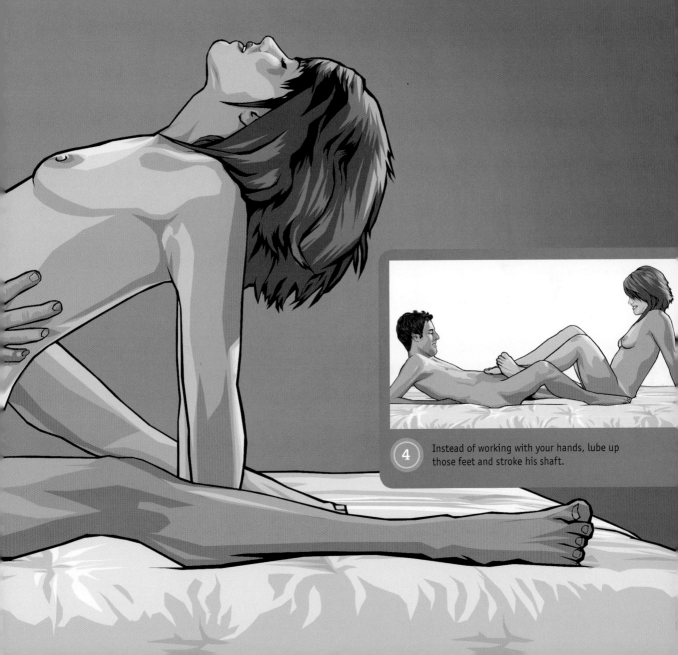

(4) Instead of working with your hands, lube up those feet and stroke his shaft.

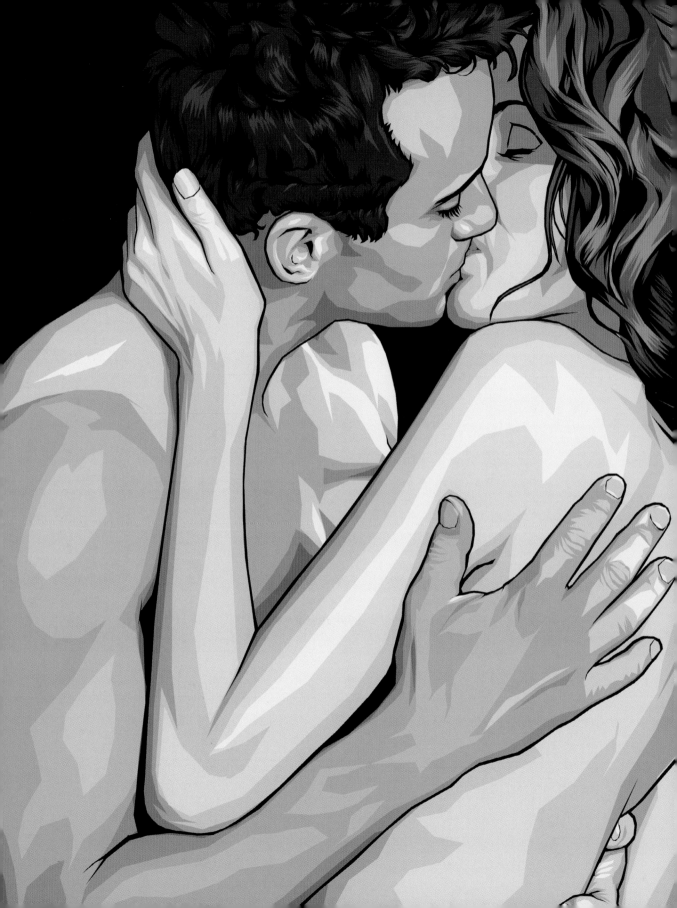

Sometimes, once we get hot and heavy, we forget that a gentle embrace or passionate kiss in the middle of wild sex can make everything feel more intense.

IT'S IN YOUR KISS (43)

One of the deepest and most powerful connections is also one of the simplest— the kiss. So intensify your lovemaking with occasional or ongoing mini make-out sessions. Start slowly, then go deep. Nibble on the upper lip, then the lower one. Or just use your lips and tongue.

Try starting with your mouths barely open, lips soft and inviting. Then move to flicking tongues quickly into each other's mouths, followed by full-on deep tongue kissing. Try sucking on your partner's lips or tongue for some variety.

You can also play with your breath. Suck some air from your partner's mouth and then gently blow it back. As you kiss, cup your lover's face, rub the back of the neck, or tug gently on a handful of their hair. Pull your partner in close, and kiss like you really mean it.

Slowly press your bodies together, letting the passion of your kiss guide your rhythm. There are so many ways to kiss, from the soft and tender to the downright animalistic. Try them all, and see what feels best to you.

44

UNCOVER HIS HOT SPOTS

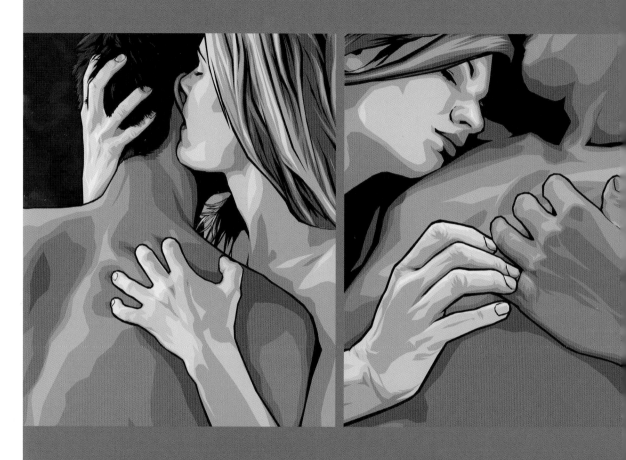

1 **HEAD GAMES** Draw him in close and nibble on his neck. Dig your nails into his back or massage his scalp. Whisper something devilish in his ear. If words get in the way, just use your tongue to flick and lick.

2 **FINGER PLAY** Use your hands (and mouth) to tantalize him. Massage his knuckles, lick along the crevices of his hands, and fool around with his fingers the same way you would with other erogenous zones.

YOUR TOUCH CAN BE TEASING OR FIRM—HE'LL LOVE IT WHEN YOU GET PRIMAL.

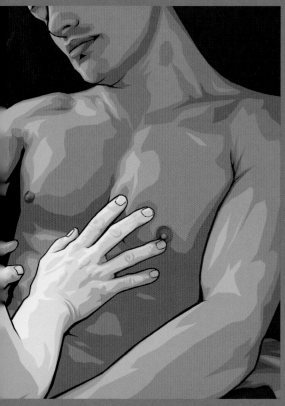

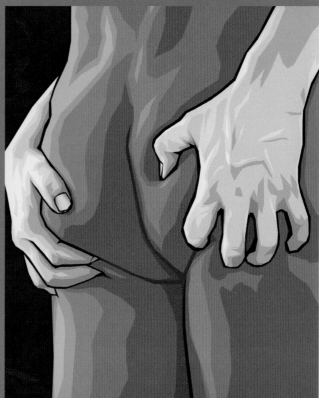

3 **TREASURE CHEST** His chest is an often-overlooked hot spot, so surprise him with a sensual chest rub. Stroke the center of his chest, and gently tease around his nipples, working up to a few playful pinches.

4 **REAR VIEW** Stroke that tantalizing rear, then give it a good, firm grab and pull his body close to yours. Breathe on his neck and kiss his shoulders. You're in charge here, so do it like you mean it. Give his butt a playful slap.

45

A TREAT FOR THE EYES

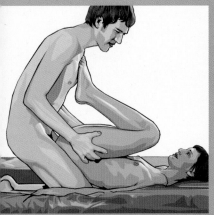

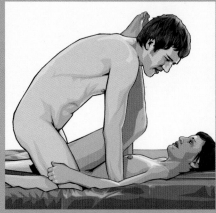

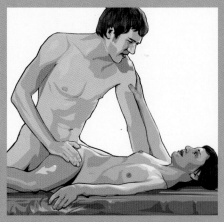

1 When her thighs are pressed together, she feels tighter, and he doesn't go in as deep.

2 For deeper penetration, she can hook heels over his shoulder and draw him in close with her feet.

3 If you're rolling over between front and rear penetration, stop midway and explore the sideways sensation.

Why do we love doggie-style sex? Well, for starters, it offers the deepest penetration, leaves his hands free to roam over her body, and lets you enjoy that primal feeling of taking and being taken. For women, it can mean incredible G-spot stimulation. And many men enjoy the fact that it's a supercomfortable and very visual position. Depending on your mood and preferences, you can get a little rough or keep things slow and sensual. Doggie is also a great position for anal sex. Whether you're going anal or vaginal, she can use her arms to brace herself against the mattress or headboard, which facilitates deeper thrusts, or he could grab her wrists from behind, supporting her upper body, for a slightly kinky feel. For health and safety reasons, never go from anal to vaginal penetration without changing condoms.

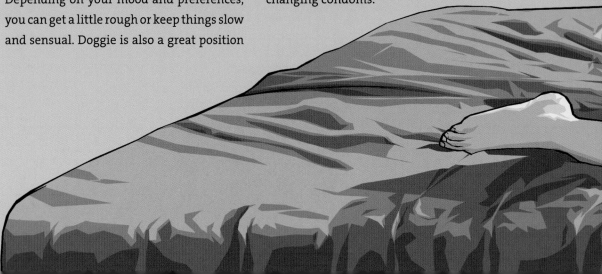

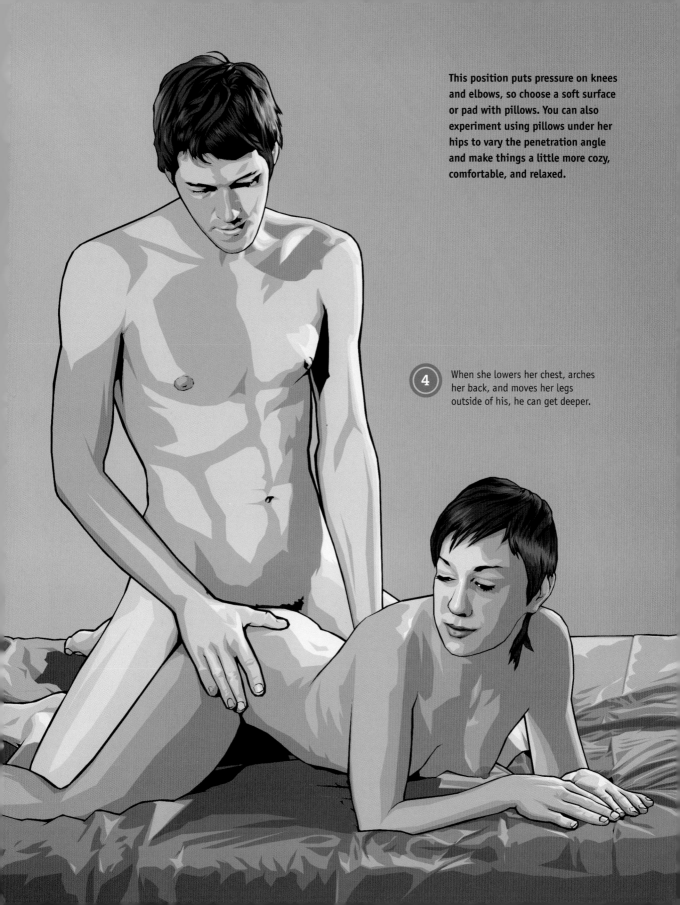

This position puts pressure on knees and elbows, so choose a soft surface or pad with pillows. You can also experiment using pillows under her hips to vary the penetration angle and make things a little more cozy, comfortable, and relaxed.

4 When she lowers her chest, arches her back, and moves her legs outside of his, he can get deeper.

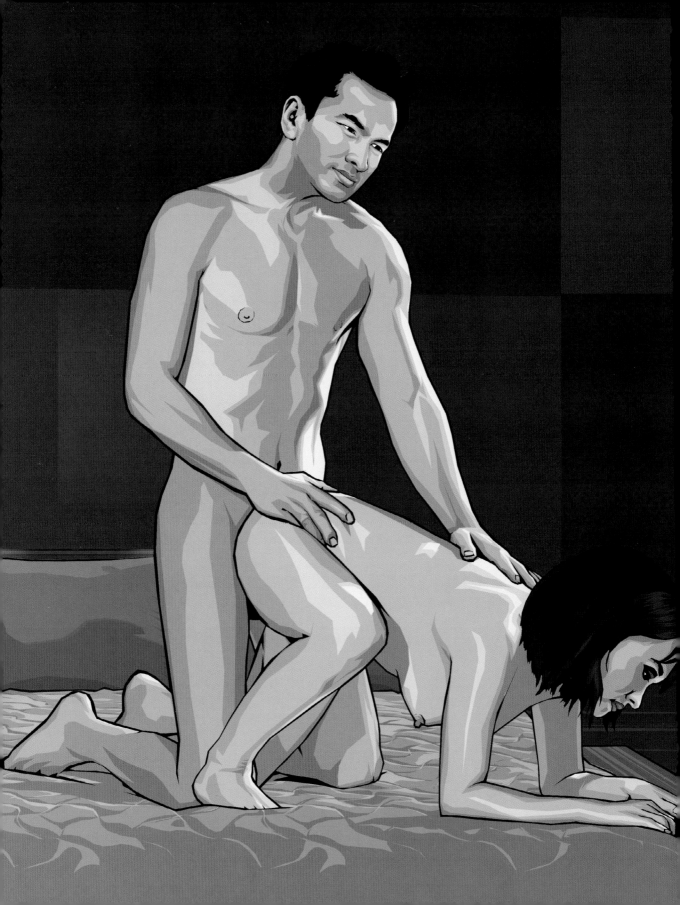

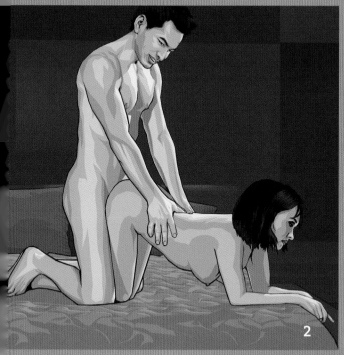

2

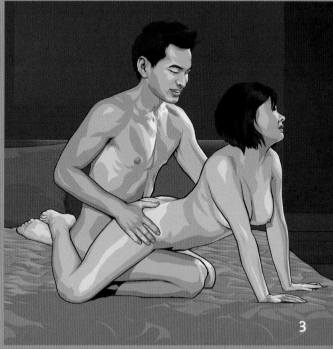

3

{1} Start with her legs in between his, and experiment with how she raises and lowers the top half of her body. Try both bent and straight arms.

{2} He can use his hands to help with the motion. When he grabs her hips, he has more power to thrust. Or he can amplify her sensations by stroking her hair, breasts, or clitoris.

{3} If she's got strong arms, he can sit back on his heels while lifting her knees and wrapping them around his body, as she slides back and forth on his body.

{4} When she's this low, she can take a break while he does the work—or she can rock into his pelvis to increase the intensity.

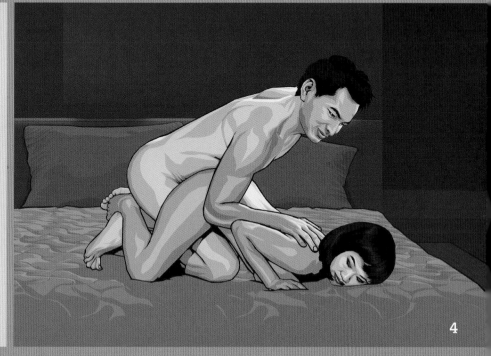

4

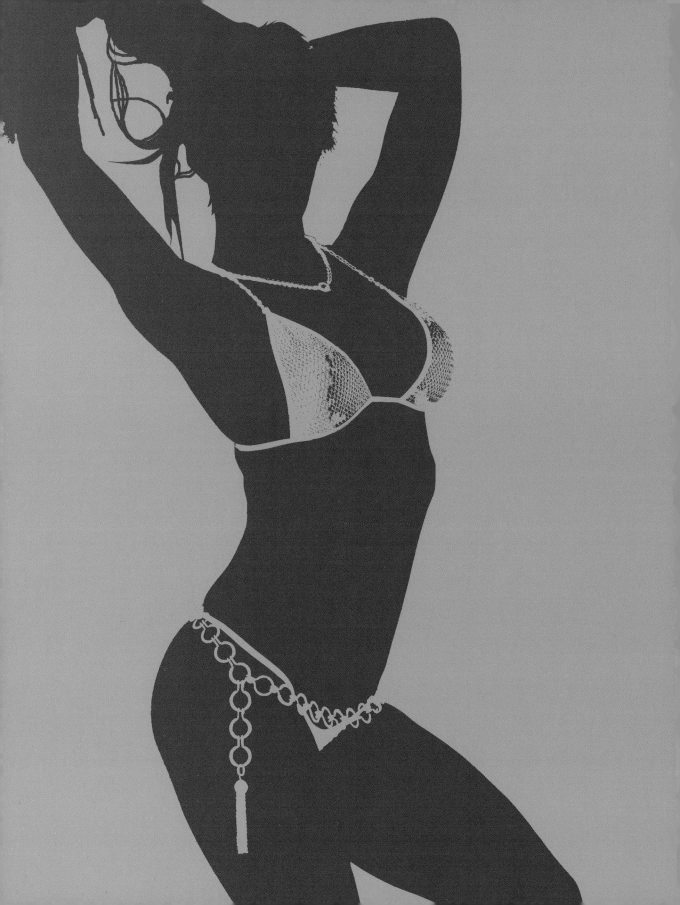

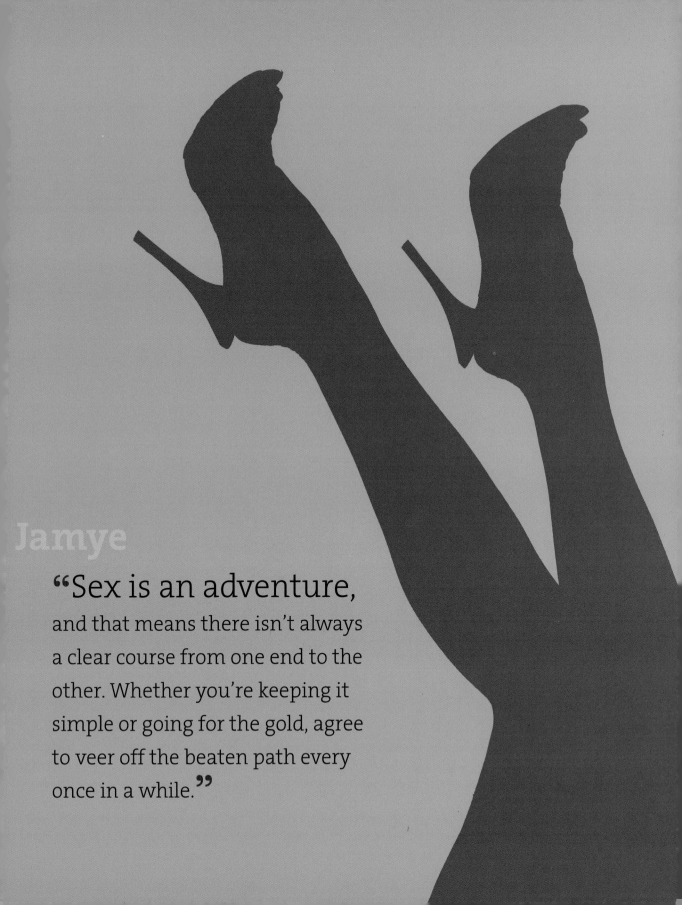

Jamye

"Sex is an adventure, and that means there isn't always a clear course from one end to the other. Whether you're keeping it simple or going for the gold, agree to veer off the beaten path every once in a while."

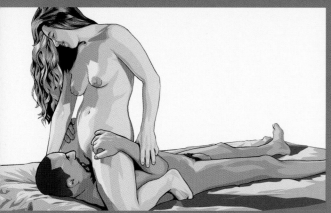

1. When she's on top, she can watch him work it. Men are famously visual, but women love sexy sights, too.

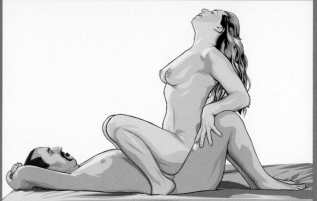

2. He can bend his legs while she squats and rides —she can push off his thighs for powerful thrusts.

3. He can guide the motion when he grabs her hips and pulls her back and forth, or he can just caress her and relish the view.

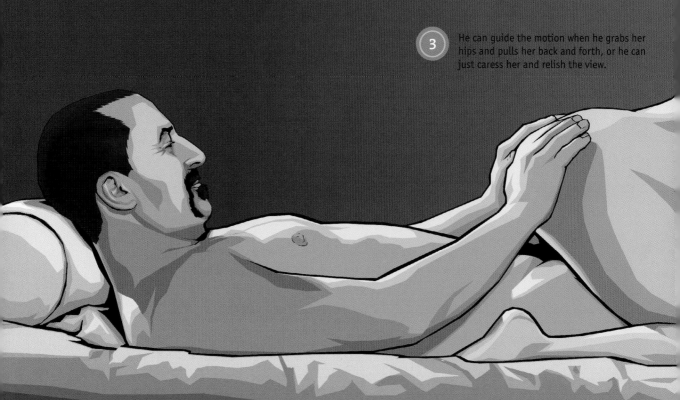

Sex in one position is fun—but swiveling sex that hits all your hot spots is even better! Reverse cowgirl, with the woman on top facing his toes, is fantastic for women who like to manage the action and men who like to admire the view. She might slip a leg in between his, or rest her stomach on his thighs. When she lies down, he gets an arresting view, and she can move her clitoris against his testicles. Shift positions carefully to make sure that the angle is comfortable for him.

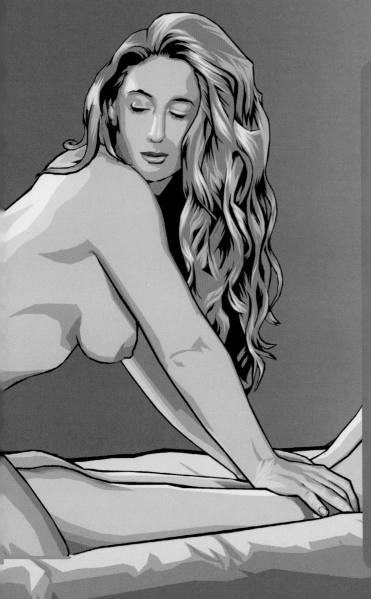

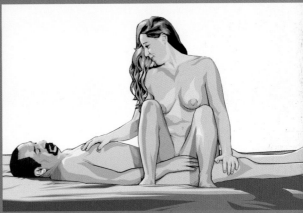

4 Swiveling slowly around while still connected is a neat trick that feels great for both of you.

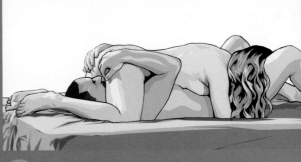

5 Once you get the rhythm, a 69 can double your oral pleasure. Try swapping who's on top.

In a seated position like this one, she's basically grinding onto his lap. If she has strong legs, she can enjoy adding a bit of up-and-down motion to the mix.

48 MAKE IT LAST ALL DAY

Some positions are all about thrusting. Others are subtler, and more about what's happening inside. Sexercise helps you get the strongest fireworks from the still, slow, and sensual positions. Squeezing and releasing your pubococcygeus (PC) muscles can increase orgasmic potential for some men and women. To locate the muscles that we're talking about, stop your flow of urine the next time you're on the toilet. The same muscles that you use to control that movement are the ones to target. Practice squeezing and releasing them all throughout the day, and then try it in any sex position. This may help women experience stronger orgasms and aid men in learning to have multiple orgasms. The key concept here is that pleasure and ejaculation are not inextricably linked. With practice, most men can learn to identify the sensations leading up to orgasm—their particular point of no return—and squeeze the PC muscle before they reach it. This allows them to stay hard and keep going until they decide to let go all the way.

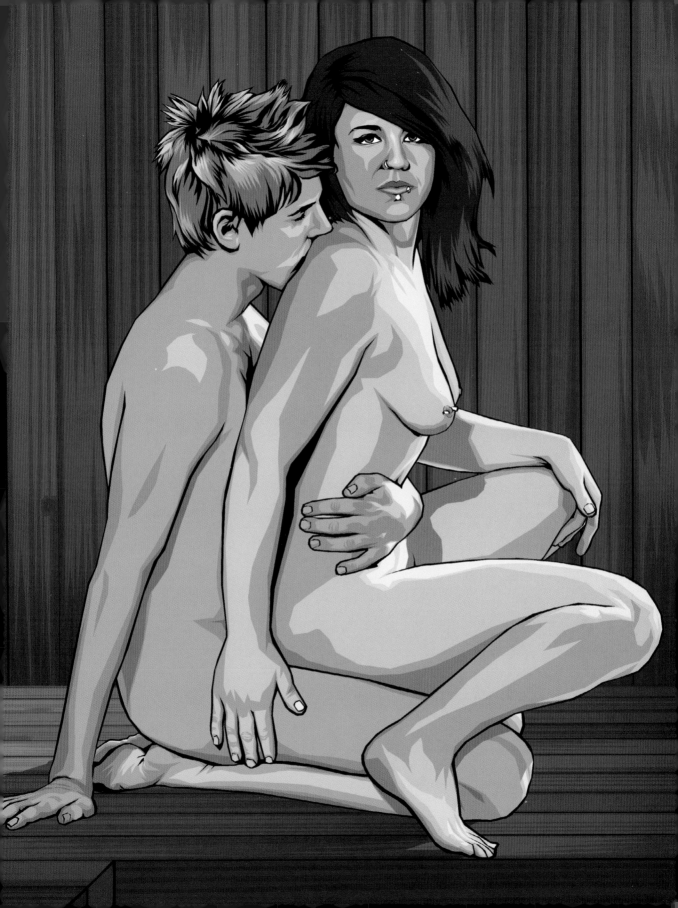

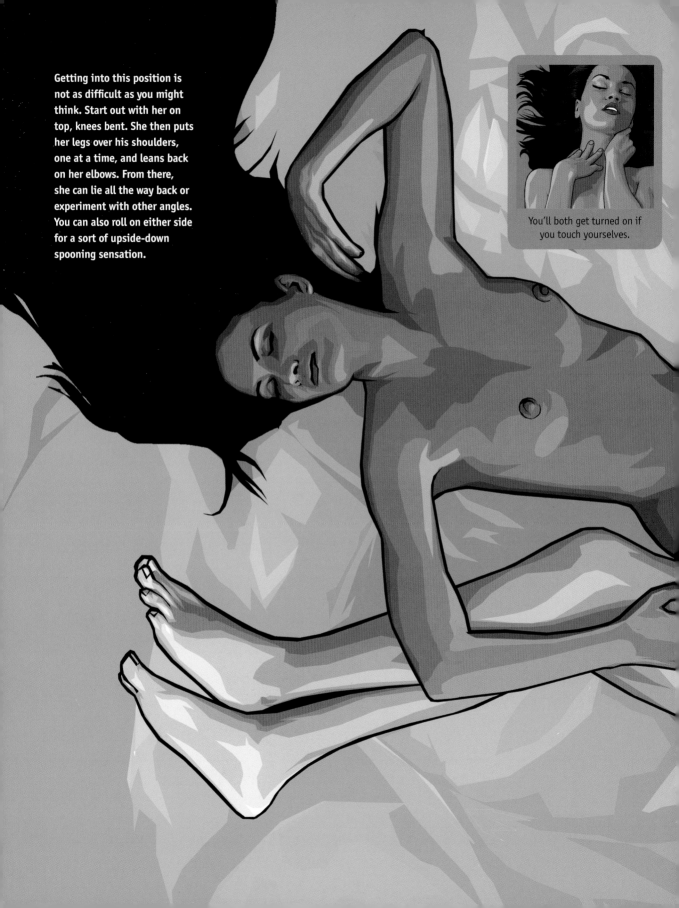

Getting into this position is not as difficult as you might think. Start out with her on top, knees bent. She then puts her legs over his shoulders, one at a time, and leans back on her elbows. From there, she can lie all the way back or experiment with other angles. You can also roll on either side for a sort of upside-down spooning sensation.

You'll both get turned on if you touch yourselves.

HEAD OVER HEELS

Not your traditional sex position, this is great for sensual, take-your-time, face-to-feet action. Because it limits eye contact, this tactic allows you to focus on touch. Use hands all over your lover's body. Tickle her clitoris, rub his feet, massage the inner thighs. Enjoy the angle, too, because this hits spots in her that she may never have felt before.

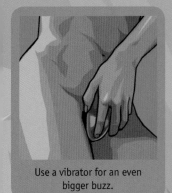

Use a vibrator for an even bigger buzz.

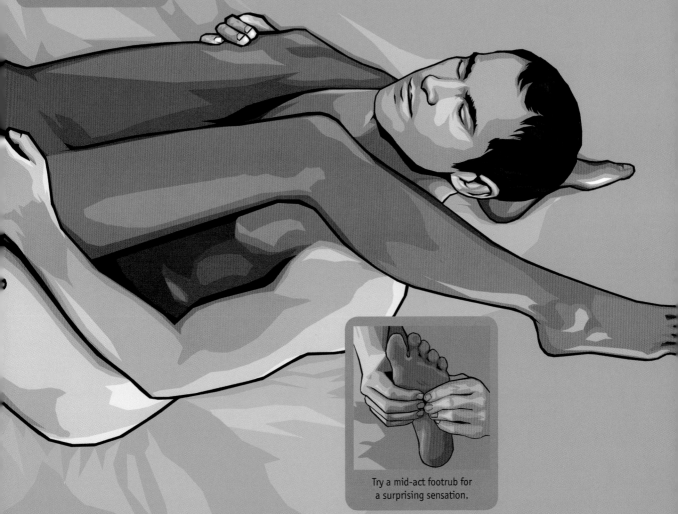

Try a mid-act footrub for a surprising sensation.

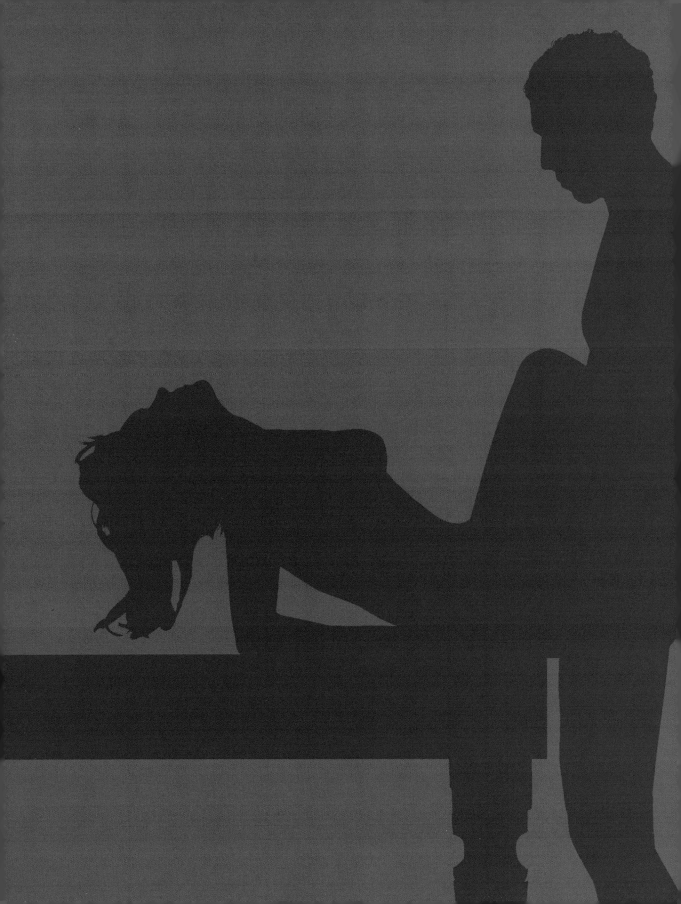

Jamye

"The shower can be a place for superb sexual contact, whether you're using it for warm-up, rubdown, or as center stage for the main event. Shower nozzles aren't just for cleaning off, they can act like a vibrator—if you can detach the head it can rock her clitoris—or if you're big into water fights, you can angle the nozzle to spray your partner all over. Getting silly in the water can throw some extra splash into your sex life."

Emily

"Spontaneous sex truly gets the adrenaline flowing. Just like in life, the unplanned events are often the ones we remember the most. So, just start with the kitchen table. And while you're in the kitchen, why even finish the meal if you can make sex the main course?"

The washing machine is ideal for adding a thrill to many positions. The height's just right, and the novelty and vibrations make for a mighty sexy combination.

50 SIT AND SPIN (CYCLE)

It might sound odd at first, but the laundry room is the perfect place to get down and dirty. The wash cycle produces an intriguing range of vibrations, and the dryer releases sensual heat—although you may want to leave the dryer off and just make your own heat. The machine doesn't even have to be turned on, as long as you both are. But when it is, you're in for a new sexual adventure.

If your heights don't quite match up, you can step on a stool or other sturdy object to help even things out a bit. In a number of positions, the woman will be the one sitting or lying on the machine, but it's also fun to try things with the guy sitting on top of it. She can then sit on him and wrap her legs around his waist, or squat over him. As the vibrations of the washing machine work their way through, it will turn him into her very own lovely vibrating sex toy.

Do a warm wash or even a hot one. If you use the cotton cycle, you'll feel the longest, fastest spin—which, of course, means the most vibration.

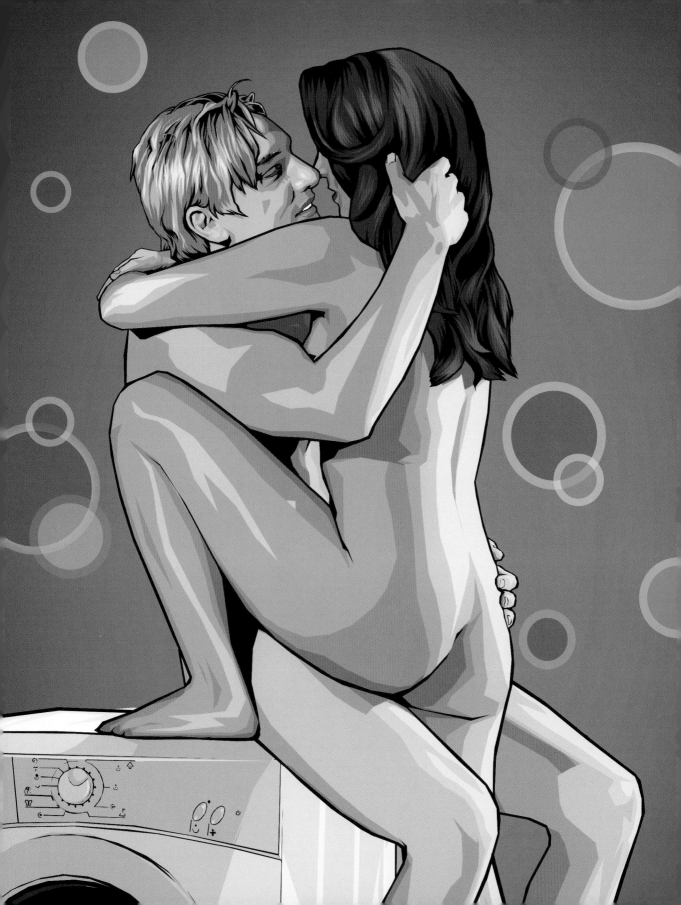

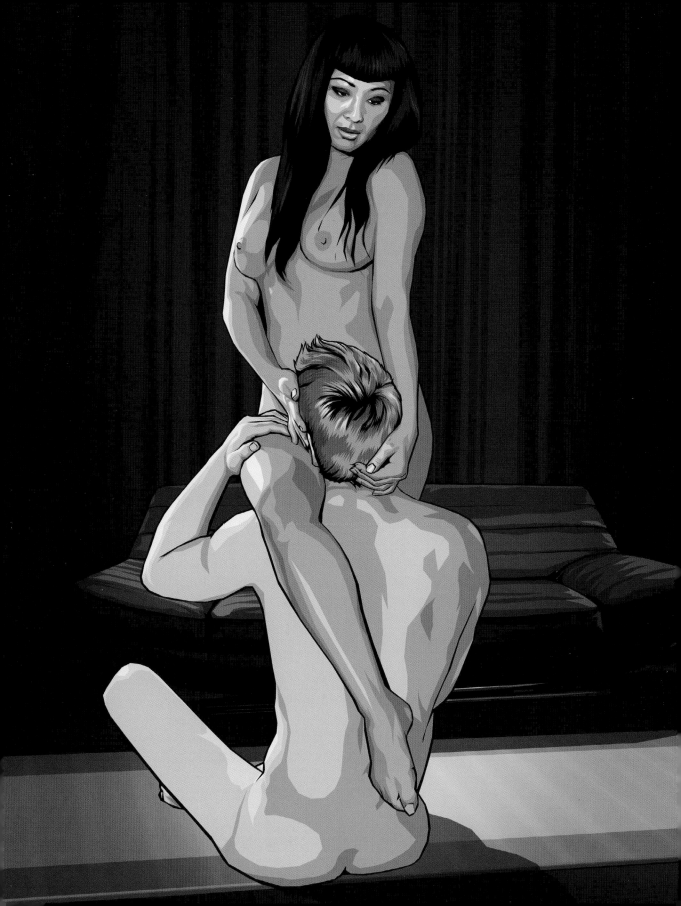

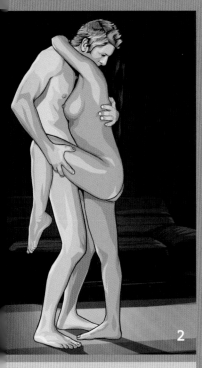

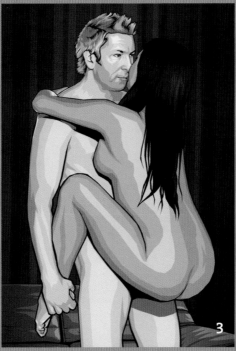

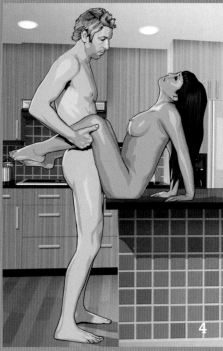

{1} Get started by warming up your lover with a little oral action.

{2} Before she jumps into your arms, have her lift one knee up.

{3} She'll be easier to lift with her arms wrapped around your shoulders. You can help support her by holding her feet, thighs, or butt.

{4} Most kitchen counters are a perfect height for this position.

{5} Alternate with her lying first on one side, then the other. You can use her shoulders for support while you thrust.

{6} End in doggie-style. Her body tucked in a tight ball will provide fabulous friction for both parties.

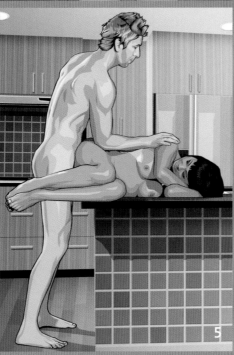

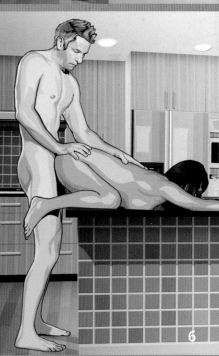

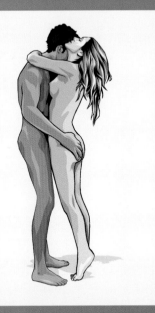

1 Don't be shy—get a little closer. Explore your partner with lips and hands to build arousal.

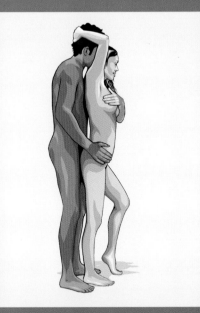

2 Work the frottage. (In layperson's terms, that means rubbing on your partner for erotic titillation.)

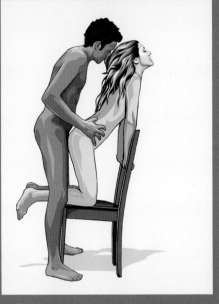

3 She can brace her body against a chair to create more resistance, which leads to deeper thrusting.

The next time you're feeling frisky, look around the house for inspiration. You can have fun with a chair, a couch, the stairs, or the dining room rug. No matter where you stage the main event, you'll find a range of ways to vary your body positions. Change who's on top and who's working harder. Try positions where you sit, stand, and spoon to benefit from all possible angles, and don't stop kissing and touching throughout—it will keep you feeling emotionally connected in the more technically challenging poses. If something feels more silly than sexy, move on. No matter where or how you do it, do it with a smile, a laugh, and love in your eyes. The best sex positions are those you enjoy with someone you feel really connected to. One safety note—be sure any chair you use is sturdy, or braced against a wall. Toppling over mid-act is no fun.

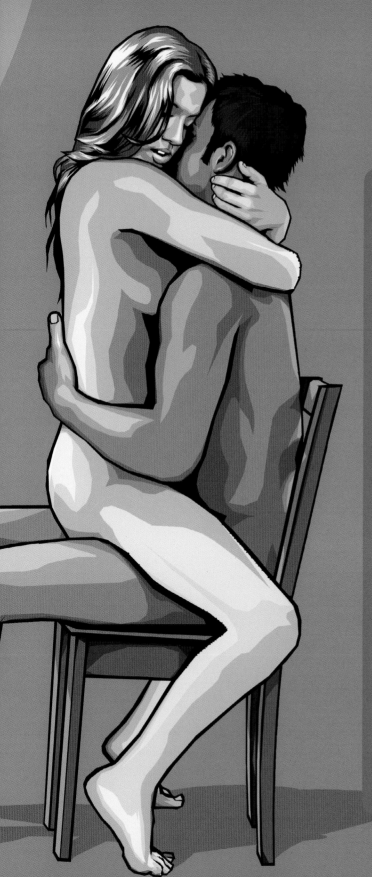

In a marathon session, take occasional breaks to help delay orgasm, increase excitement, and keep the tension mounting. The longer you last, the more fun you can have along the way.

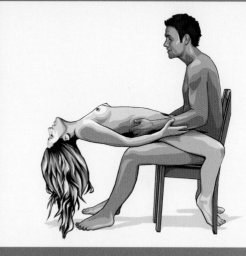

4 Even if you can't hold a position forever, don't be afraid to try new angles for experimentation.

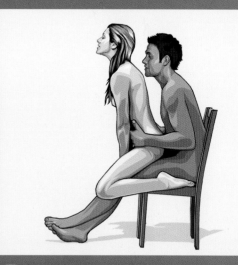

5 Turn around and around, letting your partner see the sights from all different angles.

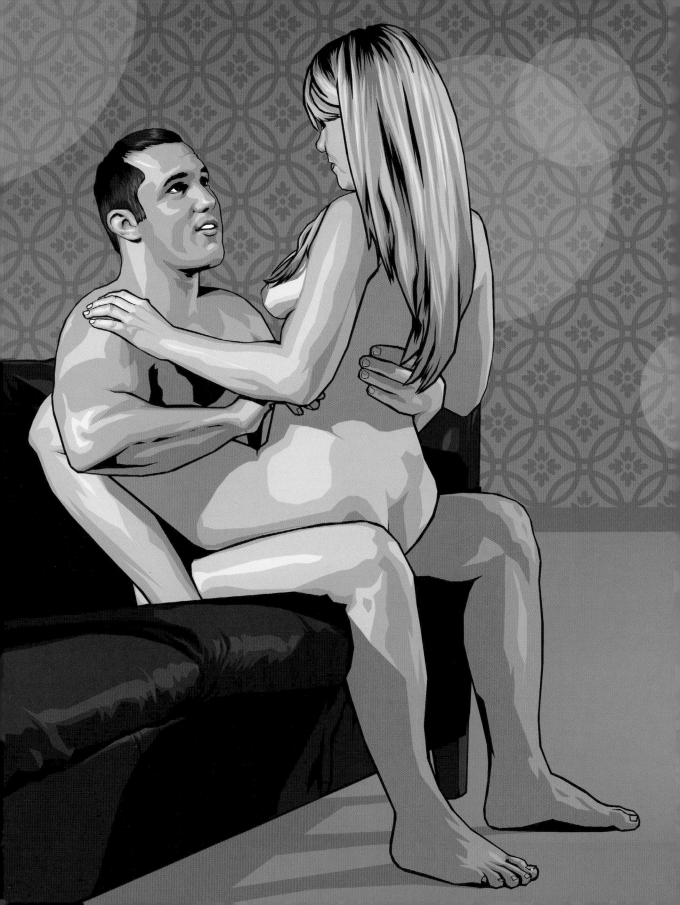

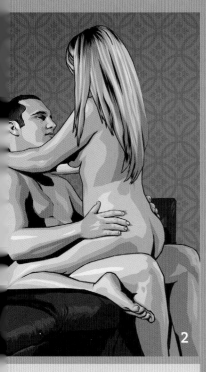

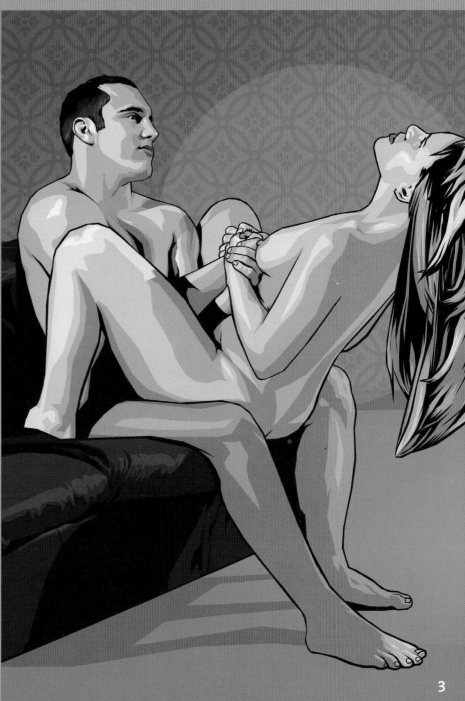

{1} As you're scouting for sexual adventure, don't overlook couches and overstuffed chairs. Comfy and casual, they provide additional back support, and their low height (compared with a bed) makes a range of sexual positions possible.

{2} The woman can straddle the man's lap; the soft, padded sofa cushions might make riding easier on her knees. If the cushions aren't cooperating, he can bounce his knees a bit, sending her up and down with hardly any effort.

{3} Hold hands so she can lean back farther—this creates an anchoring line that allows for heavier rocking and rolling.

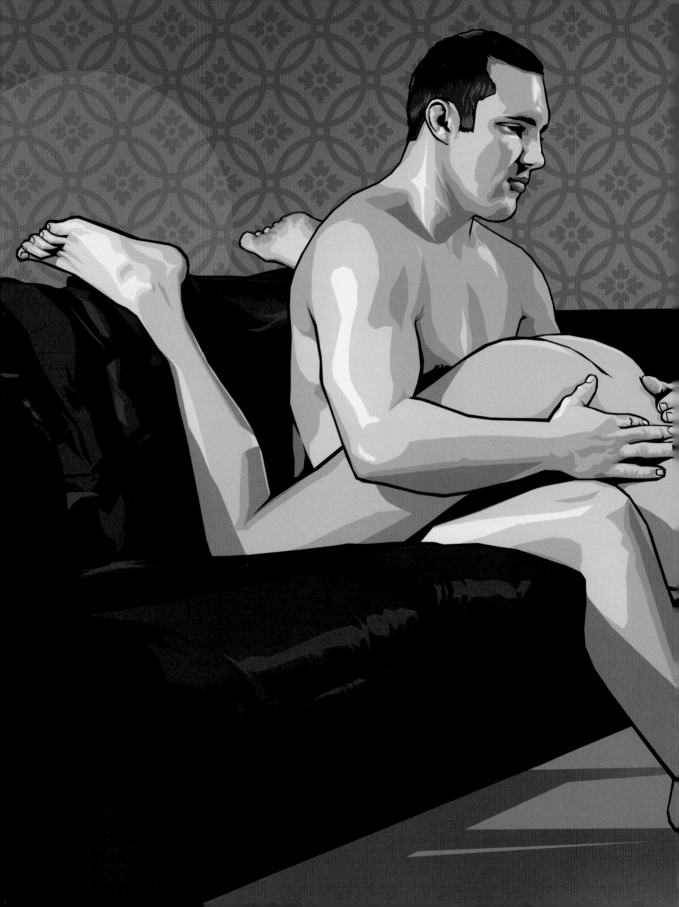

FOUR ON THE FLOOR

You may have seen a standing wheelbarrow position depicted in books or movies—the man standing, penetrating the woman while she walks on her hands. It looks interesting, but it's neither easy to do nor particularly satisfying. Instead of going to extremes, try this alternative wheelbarrow instead.

To get in this position, she starts in reverse cowgirl, then slowly leans forward so that her hands rest on the floor.

For an especially adventurous and athletic variation, start out facing each other, with the woman on top. She then slowly arches back until her hands hit the floor behind her in a bridge-like stance. With her hands on the floor for support, she'll be able to thrust herself up and down on his body.

If you're looking for a place to get away (whether from the family, roommates, or just from the bed), the shower is a delightful alternative to sex on dry land.

55 GET DIRTY IN THE SHOWER

The shower is tailor-made for steamy sex sessions. It's warm, it's wet, and it lets you go wild, since the sound of running water drowns out any squeals, grunts, or groans you might make.

A position with the woman bending over and the man entering her from behind works wonderfully in the shower. It offers stability, because she can anchor her hands on her calves for support. (This pose is also great for sex anywhere you don't have a good surface to lean on.) If you're more of a bathtub couple, climb on in there—bubbles add some soapy fun. He can recline in the tub while she crouches above him, grabbing on to the tub's side for a little extra stability.

Whether you're doing it in the shower or in the bathtub, you'll want to use a silicone-based lubricant. Silicone lubes are waterproof, meaning they need both soap and water to be removed and won't wash off unless you want them to. Do be sure to rinse all your bits before you leave the shower—you're already in there, so you may as well get clean!

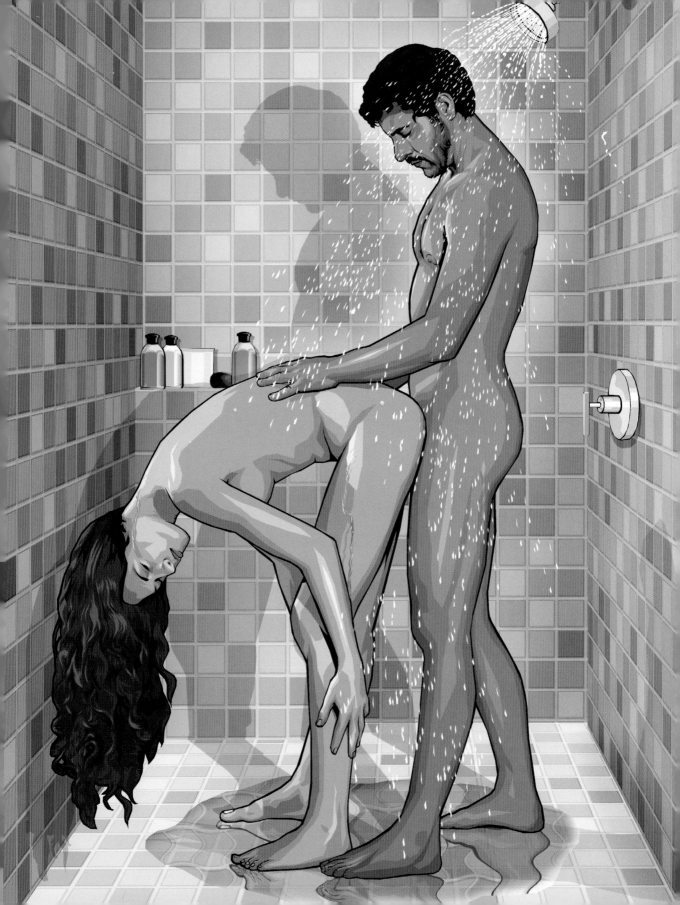

56

ALL OVER THE HOUSE

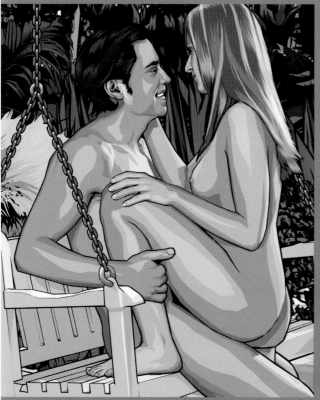

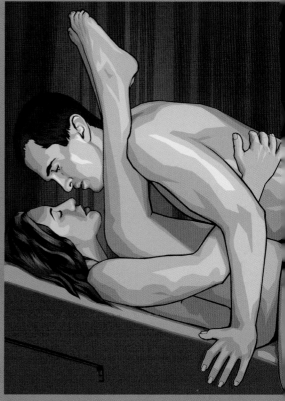

SWINGING ON THE PORCH A swing on the porch, a poolside lounge, or other garden furniture lets you experience outdoor action without fear of prying eyes. Just be sure your neighbors don't have a view into your yard.

PILLOW PROPS Pillows allow you to try a range of positions and angles that might otherwise be uncomfortable. And a pillow placed under a woman's lower back during missionary sex provides more direct clitoral stimulation.

LOOK WITH THE RIGHT EYES, AND EVERY SURFACE IN YOUR HOUSE SEEMS SEXY.

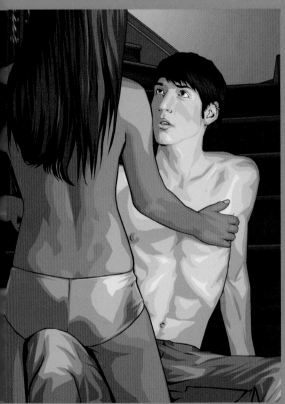 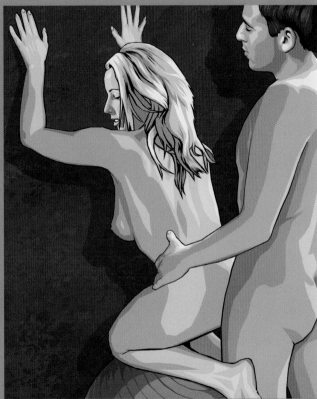

STEP IT UP Want it so bad you can't even make it upstairs? It can be wildly sexy to just strip down and do it right there. She can push him onto the steps and ride him, or he can bend her over the first step and take her from behind.

HAVE A BALL A Pilates ball can be used for more than one kind of workout. She can kneel on it, braced against a wall; lie with her back on the ball and her knees bent; or bend over it. Just keep the action gentle so you don't lose your balance.

57

THE LOOK OF LOVE

This stance allows you to make sexy eye contact and relish the full sight of each other's naked bodies. With her feet over his shoulders, he can feel himself deep inside her, while she controls the speed of thrusting. Or she may choose to lie flat on her back and wrap her legs around his waist.

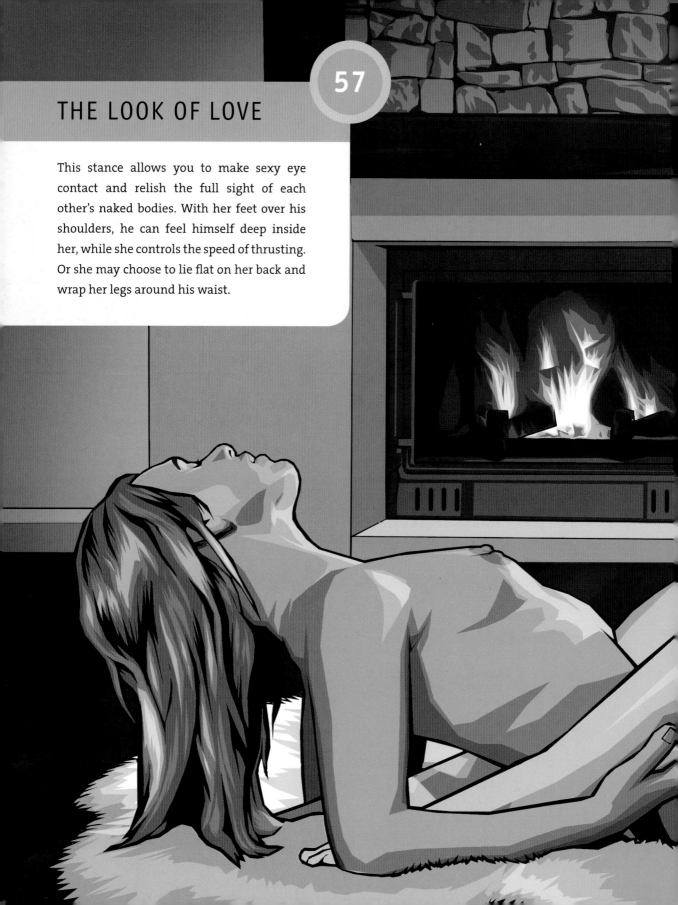

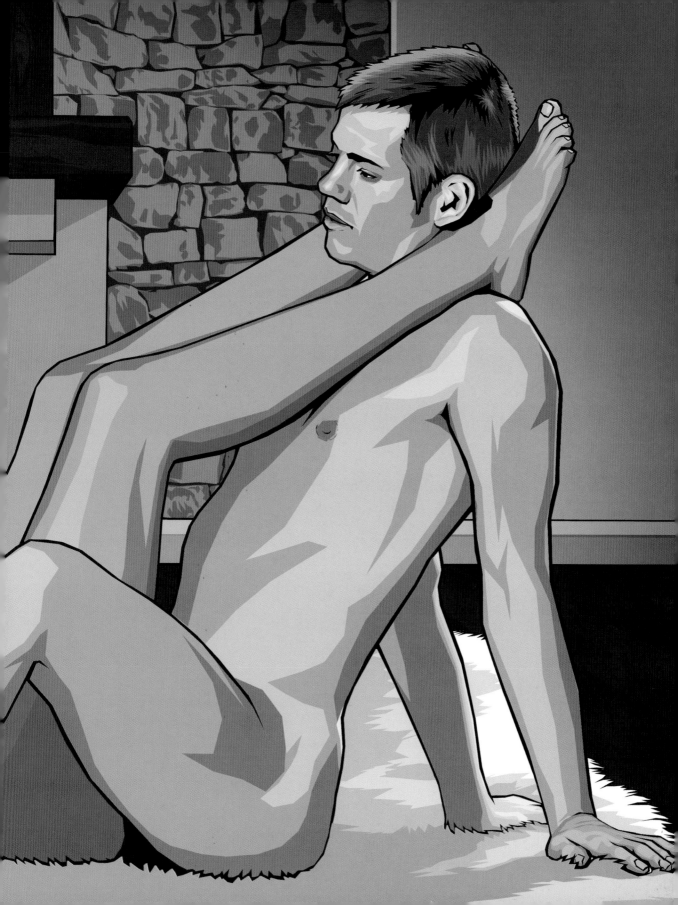

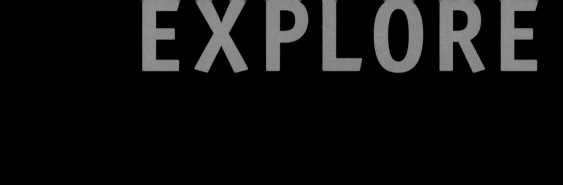
EXPLORE

Communication is truly the key to an adventurous and satisfying sex life. **Is adventure necessary?** Maybe not for everyone, but most people get a little tired of eating the same foods or having the same conversations every day. The same goes for having the same sex. Talk about the sex you're having right now and the sex you'd like to have. Discuss your desires and your limits, decide what you'd like to do together, and check in with each other while you explore your boundaries. To get the conversation started, we've given a range of ideas from bondage to spanking and from tantric sex to threesomes. We're not suggesting you try them all, at least not yet. You should never feel pressured to do anything you don't want to, and you can decide anytime that what you're doing isn't working for you. What we do hope is that these ideas will spark your sexual creativity and help you create the sex life you've dreamed of.

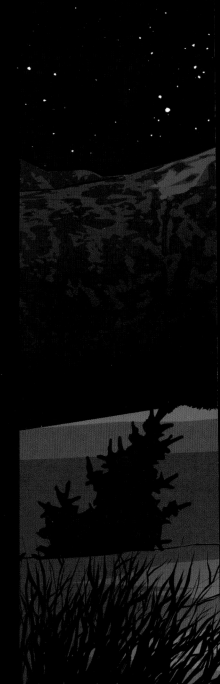

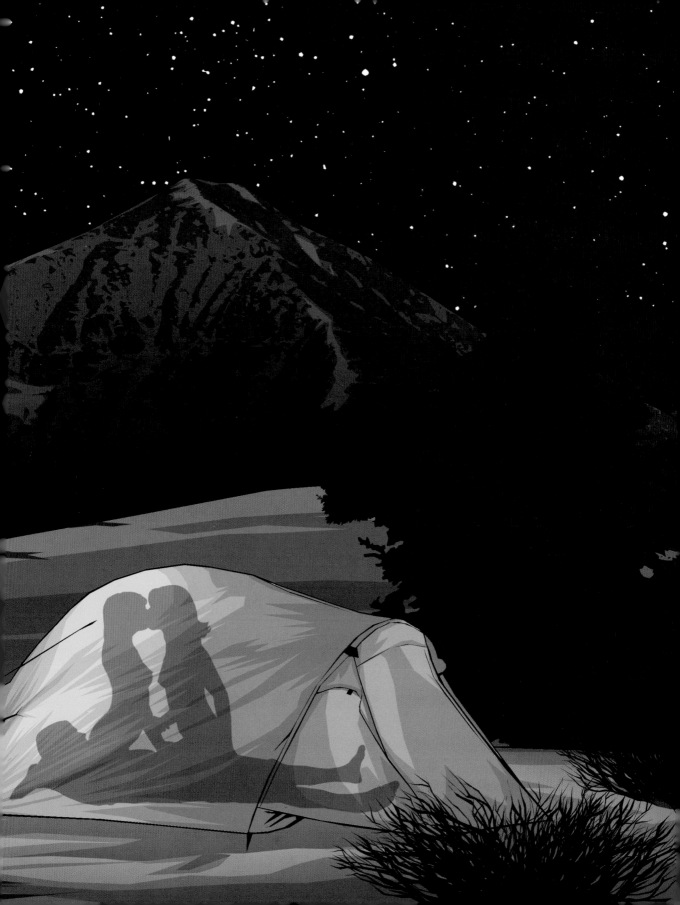

Bondage describes any sexual situation in which a person is restrained. It may involve a scarf, cuffs, or rope. You can even restrain a partner with your voice alone.

58 BONDAGE 101

Start slowly, with gentle touches. Stroke your partner's hair and back, then move on. Ask your partner if he or she will submit to you. Wait for a yes, then slowly and sensually lower him or her down to the floor, mattress, or chair. First try holding your partner's hands down with your body, or restrain his or her hands above the head, in front of the chest, or behind the back. Or tie the hands together or to a piece of furniture like the headboard. You can also play with bondage using nothing but words. Put your partner in a spot or position that appeals to you and order him or her to stay still. Start pleasuring your partner and, if he or she moves, stop, gaze into his or her eyes, and say, "I told you not to move!" Then tell your partner that you'll only do what you're told. Make them express their desires in exquisite detail.

Although one of you might feel more comfortable as the "top" and the other as the "bottom" during these games, you might want to try switching things up, just to see how the other half feels.

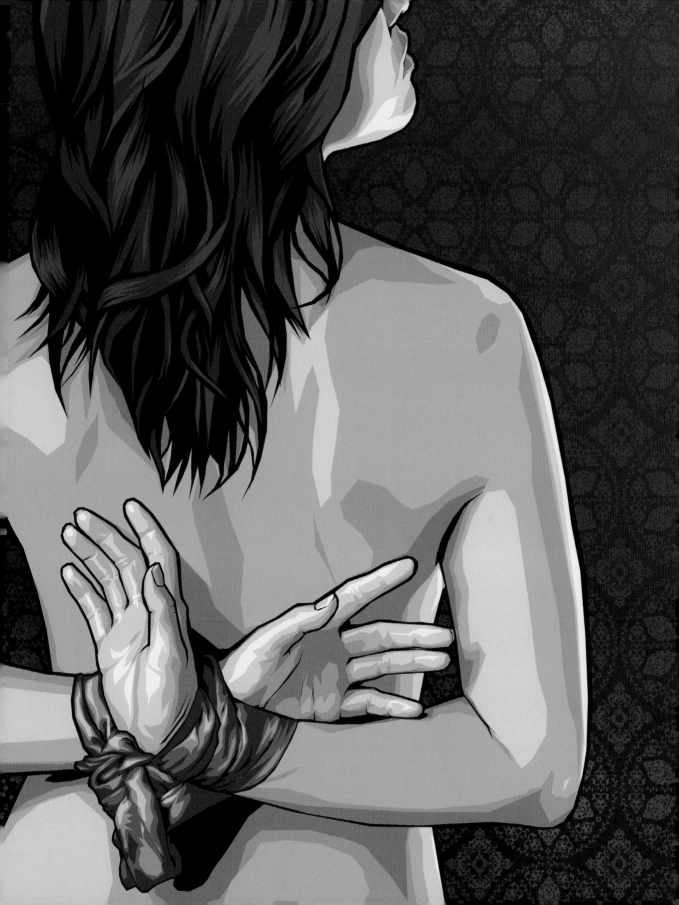

59

ALL TIED UP

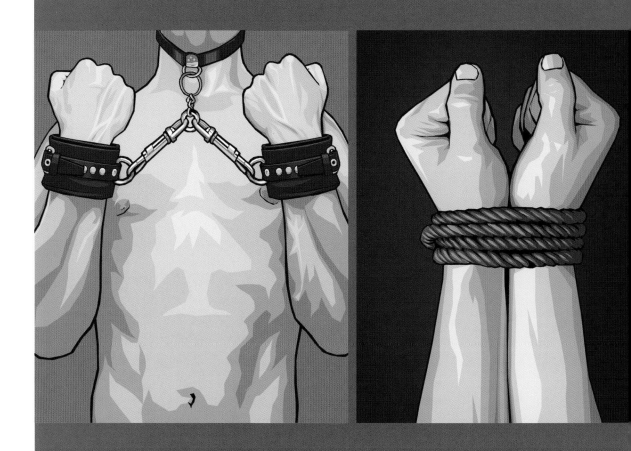

CUFFS Bondage cuffs are a quick and easy way to restrain your partner—no special knots required. They can fit the wrists, ankles, neck, and even thighs. Some are leather with hooks and loops; others are fabric with handy fastenings.

ROPE You can do a lot with rope, from the simple to the artistic, but first you'll have to choose between textures and materials, from inexpensive nylon to fancy silk. Have scissors on hand in case you can't undo your knots.

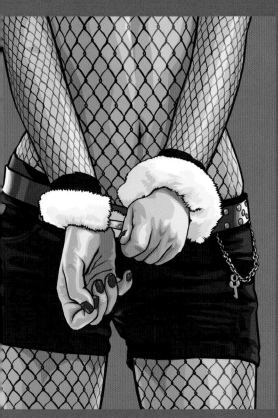

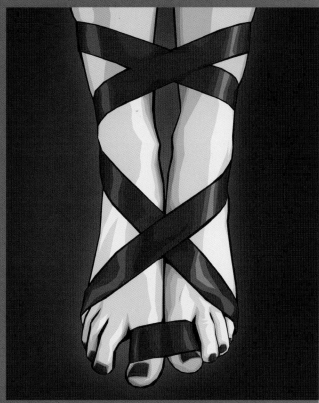

HANDCUFFS Metal handcuffs are sold in sex shops, but unless you're really into the police fantasy, you'll probably find them uncomfortable. Look for cuffs that are well padded—and be sure to have a spare key, just in case.

RIBBONS Ribbons are great for simple bondage, as they're lightweight and no one will raise an eyebrow if you leave them lying around. You can also try using bondage tape, which is sturdier and easy to adjust and remove.

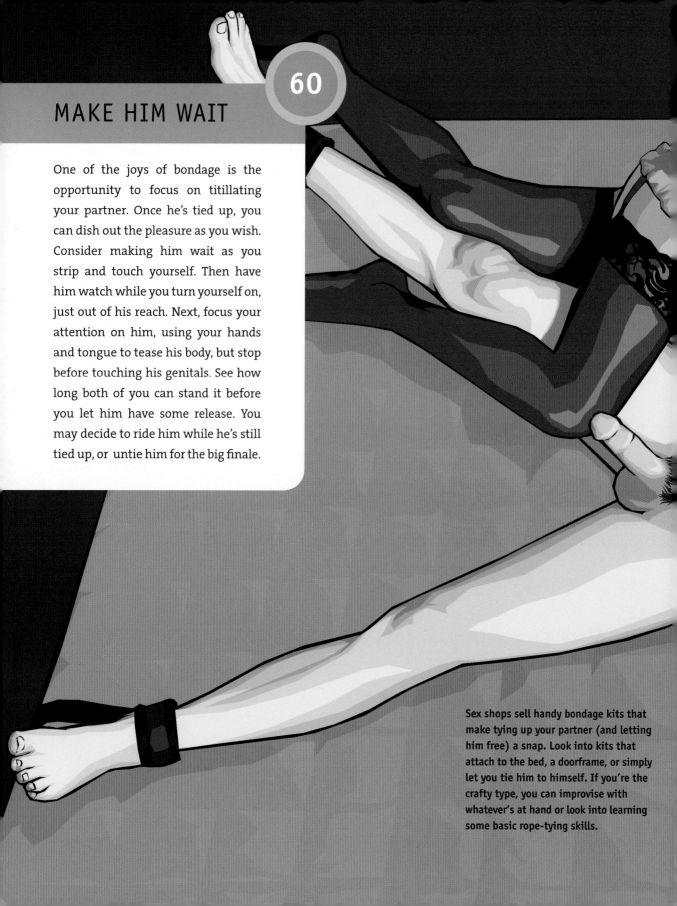

60

MAKE HIM WAIT

One of the joys of bondage is the opportunity to focus on titillating your partner. Once he's tied up, you can dish out the pleasure as you wish. Consider making him wait as you strip and touch yourself. Then have him watch while you turn yourself on, just out of his reach. Next, focus your attention on him, using your hands and tongue to tease his body, but stop before touching his genitals. See how long both of you can stand it before you let him have some release. You may decide to ride him while he's still tied up, or untie him for the big finale.

Sex shops sell handy bondage kits that make tying up your partner (and letting him free) a snap. Look into kits that attach to the bed, a doorframe, or simply let you tie him to himself. If you're the crafty type, you can improvise with whatever's at hand or look into learning some basic rope-tying skills.

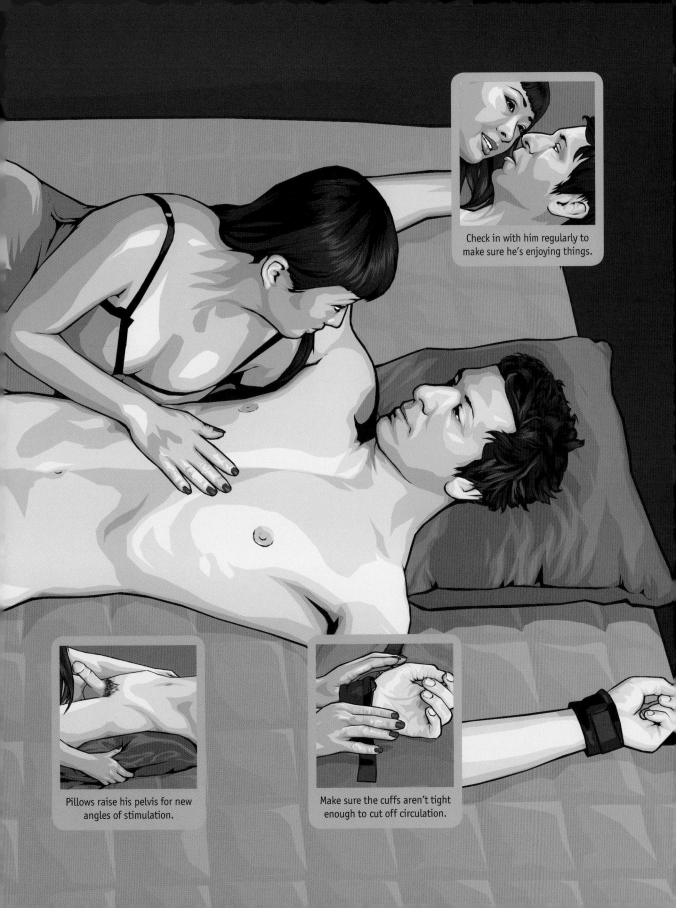

Check in with him regularly to make sure he's enjoying things.

Pillows raise his pelvis for new angles of stimulation.

Make sure the cuffs aren't tight enough to cut off circulation.

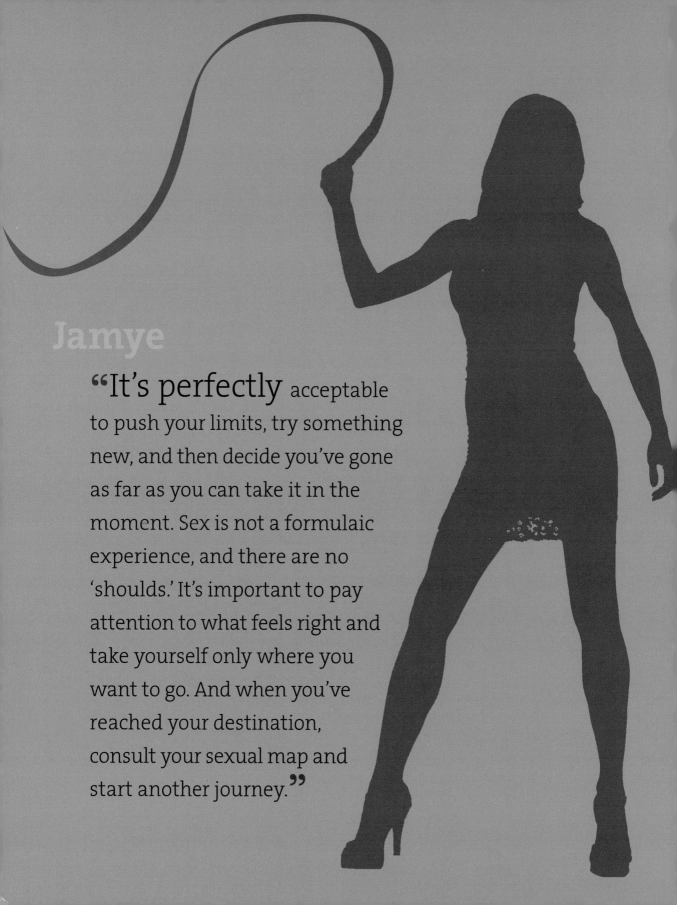

Jamye

"It's perfectly acceptable to push your limits, try something new, and then decide you've gone as far as you can take it in the moment. Sex is not a formulaic experience, and there are no 'shoulds.' It's important to pay attention to what feels right and take yourself only where you want to go. And when you've reached your destination, consult your sexual map and start another journey."

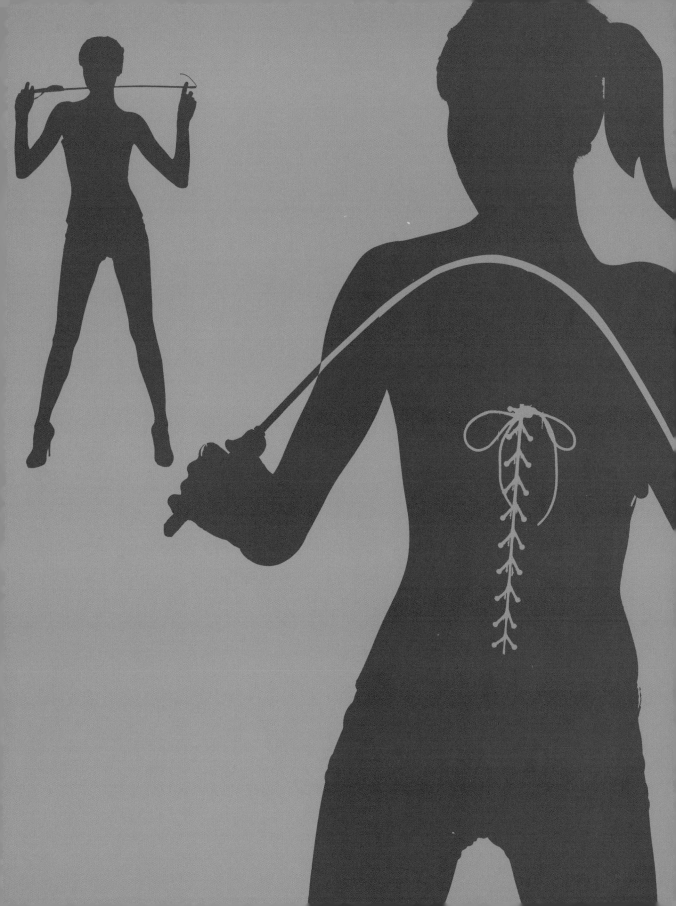

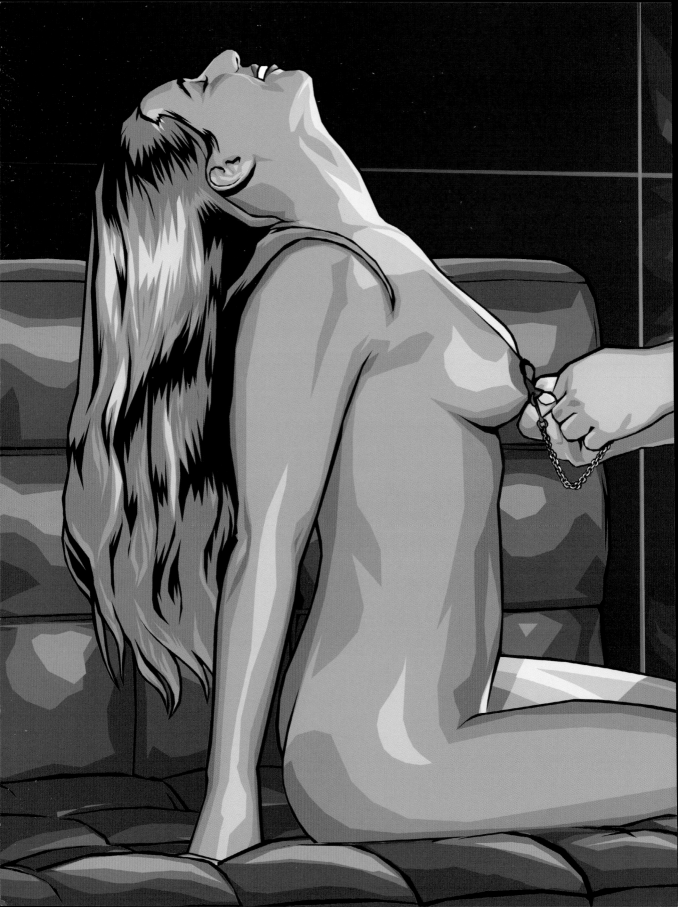

If you enjoy intense thrills, you might want to try toys and techniques that stimulate you or your partner in ways that range from subtle to extreme.

SERIOUS SENSATIONS 61

We all have our own distinct definitions of pleasure and pain, so why not learn about your own and your partner's? Try toys on yourself first, so you know how they feel before using them on your lover.

Nipple clamps have an effect when you first clip them on, when you tighten them, and when you take them off (that's actually the moment when they hurt the most). For beginners, try tweezer or crocodile clamps. Both allow you to adjust the strength, so you can go from light to "ouch!" (and back) in a heartbeat.

Clothespins are easy to find, inexpensive, and simple to apply. They can be used on the breasts, chest, and genitals for varying levels of pleasure, pain, and pleasurable pain. Plastic or metal pins tend to give a more intense sensation.

For a more subtle set of feelings, the Wartenberg wheel (aka the pinwheel) can be used for delightful and devious play. Run it over your lover's back, legs, breasts, arms, and genitals—depending on pressure, it can tickle or sting. Hold it at an angle, and don't press too hard.

A GOOD SPANKING

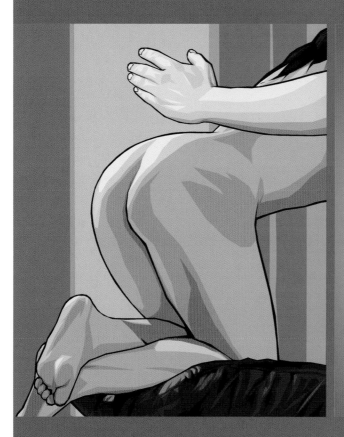

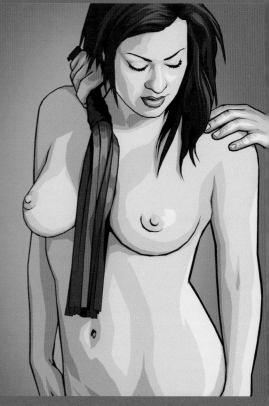

BARE-HANDED SPANK Your hand can deliver some pretty hard slaps, so start slowly, alternate butt cheeks, and check with your partner so that you're headed where you both want to go. Aim for the most padded part of the butt and thighs.

FLOGGER A flogger is made with strips of leather, rubber, or even ribbons. Trail it along your partner's chest or belly for a light tickle. If you're after more of a whipping effect, flick it against your playmate's legs, back, or buttocks.

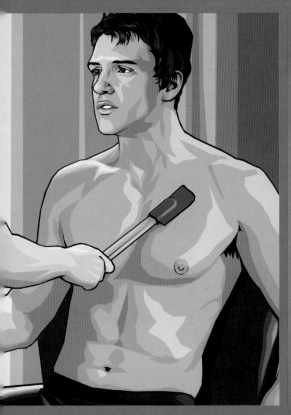

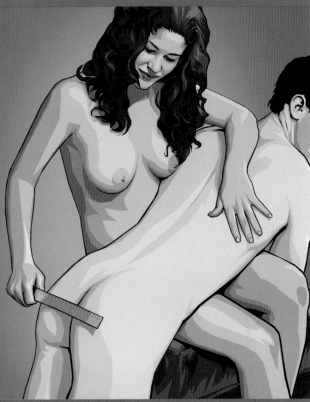

PADDLE You can find various kinds of specialty paddles in shops—or scour your home for pervertables, everyday household items that can be used for sexual play, such as ping-pong paddles, spatulas, or even a hardback book.

RULER If you get a thrill from student-teacher games, you may want to use a ruler as an extra-credit sex-cessory. It's a perfect alternative to a paddle, so why not place your lucky student over your knee and teach him or her a real lesson?

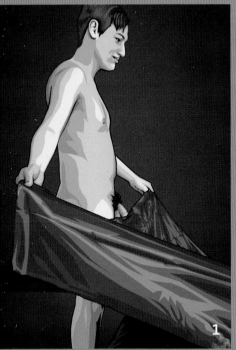

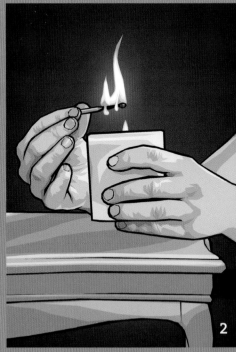

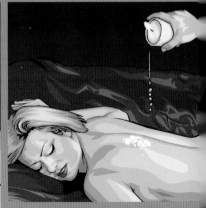

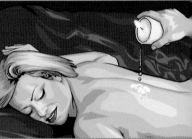

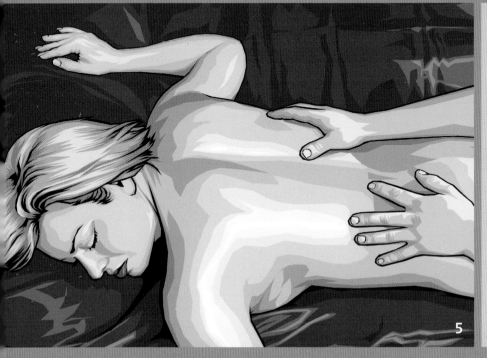

{1} Lay down a sheet or towel to protect your bedding and furniture.

{2} Use a massage candle or an unscented, plain white paraffin candle, which burns cooler.

{3} Let the wax pool. Avoid dripping wax that's just been in contact with the flame. Test the heat on your hand, then start dripping from at least 3 feet (1 m) above your partner.

{4} If she enjoys the sensation, try dripping it from a lower height for greater intensity.

{5} A massage candle's wax will turn to scented oil on your partner's skin. If you're using a regular candle, allow the wax to dry, then peel it off.

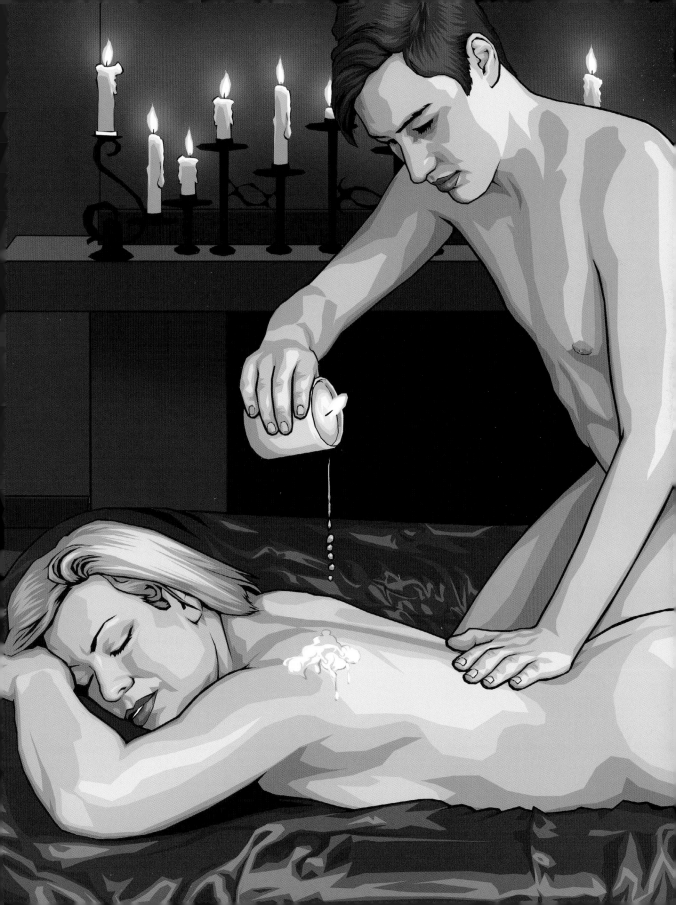

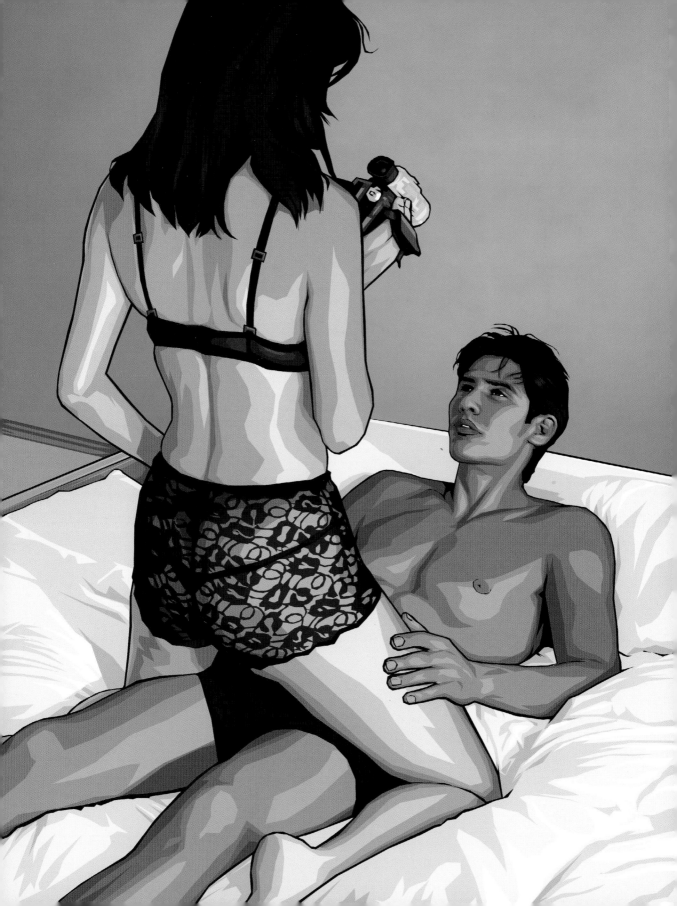

Making your own sexy video can feel both devilishly hot and a little bit daunting. Agree on a plan to keep your skin flick private, then feel free to go wild.

CAUGHT ON VIDEO 64

The first step is deciding what you want to do with your naughty movie. You may decide to erase the video after you watch it, burn it to a DVD, or save it on a flash drive that you can lock away. Then pick out your wardrobe or have your partner style you. Wear something that makes you feel sexy, whether that's a thong bikini or a long silk kimono.

Next, get the set ready: remove all the clutter and extras you don't want seen in the frame, be it dirty laundry or family pictures. You can even change the bulbs in your lamps. Purple or red lights give off a softer and more sensual look.

You can script the action but generally, the more natural you are, the better your on-screen chemistry. Many people find missionary the most flattering position, but do experiment. A microphone will capture your sexy sounds—and maybe some giggling as well.

Not every man will enjoy "backdoor" stimulation, but he won't know unless he tries it. Start gently, try a few approaches, and he may discover a new thrill or two.

65 BEHIND EVERY GOOD MAN . . .

There are a number of ways to stimulate the prostate, a man's main source of anal pleasure. You can apply pressure to the perineum, the area between the testicles and anus, to stimulate without penetration. Or use a lubricated, gloved finger or a small dildo to probe gently. When choosing a toy for anal play, it's important to pick one that has a flared base so that it can't slip all the way inside.

Strap-on sex—which is also referred to as pegging—has become more and more popular in recent years (or perhaps people are feeling increasingly empowered to talk about it). If you're wearing a harness, be sure the dildo you're using will stay securely fastened. Start with a smaller toy than you think you'll want (you can always upgrade), and go very slowly, with lots of lubrication and communication about what feels good. The man may want to masturbate or have you play with him, or just enjoy the sensations. Even if it doesn't lead to orgasm, prostate play can be a fantastic part of a rich and experimental sex life.

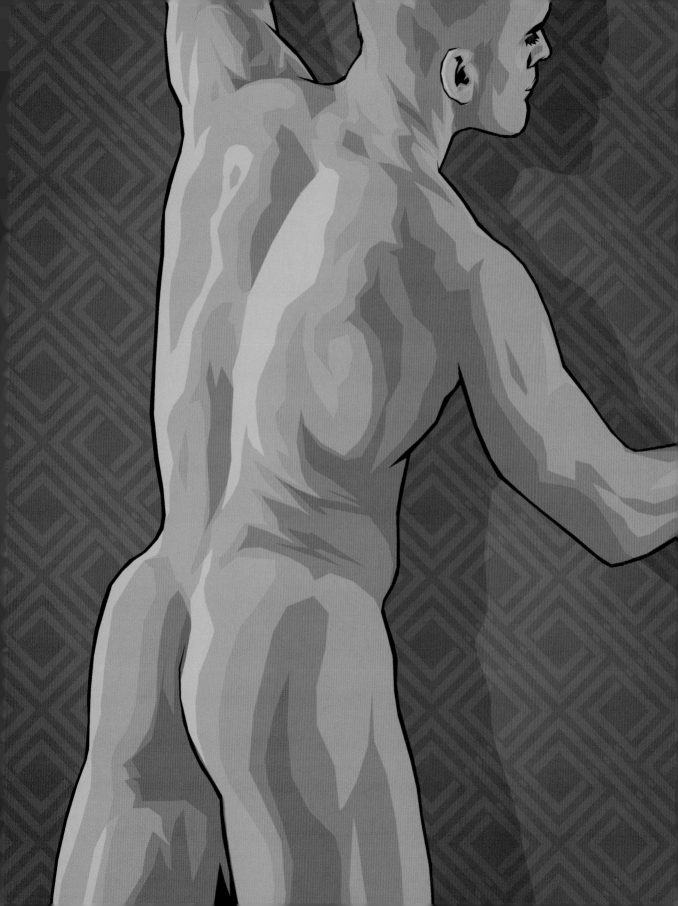

Jamye

"I like to call some of those crazy moves in sex 'porn-star acrobatics.' Porn stars are paid professionals whose job it is to get down in ways we rarely think of trying. As long as you feel safe and things are consensual, you, too, can go wild!"

Emily

"Trying new positions will exercise your sexual muscles. It's an invigorating challenge that can lead to more intense orgasms and will build your self-confidence and sexual repertoire."

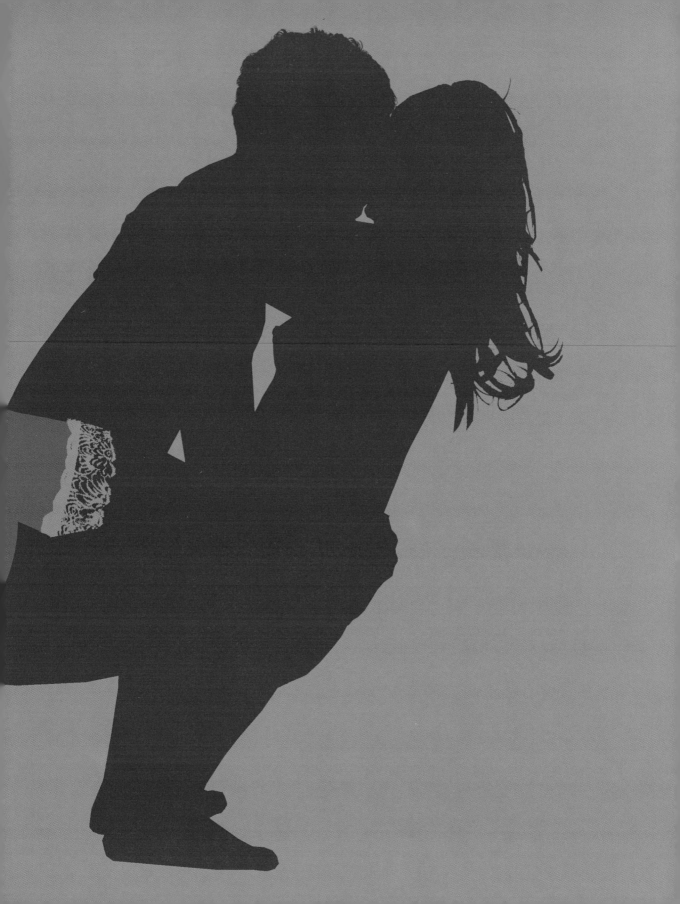

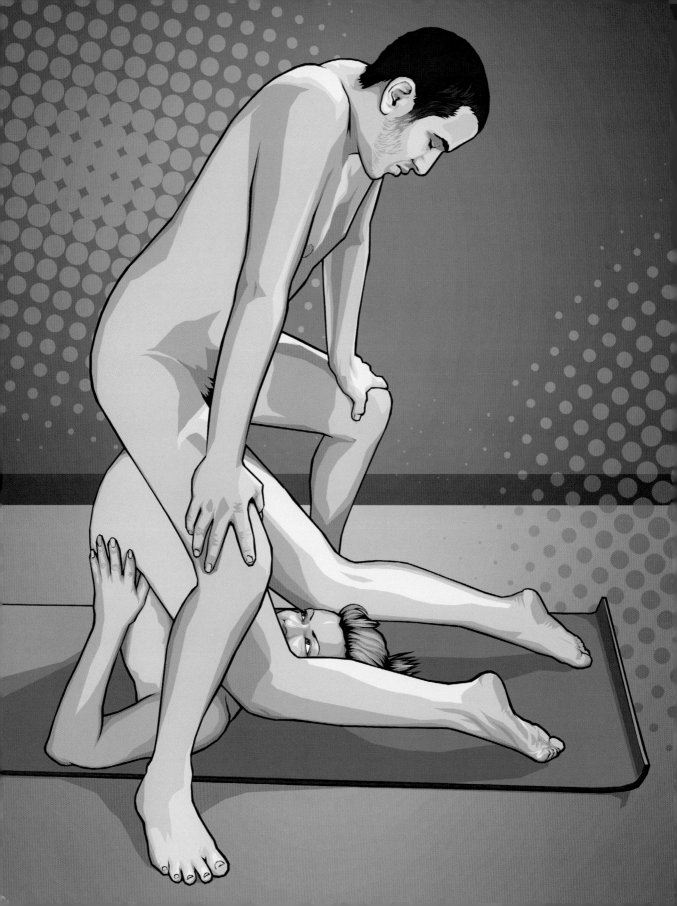

THE PILE DRIVER

This is one of those acrobatic sex positions that you might see in pornography. Much of its appeal is visual: it puts everything right out there on display for the lovers. To get into this position, the woman lies on the floor and flips her legs over her shoulders, as if she were doing a shoulder stand. Some women find it more comfortable to brace their lower back against a pillow or a piece of furniture. The man needs strong leg muscles, as he's essentially doing an extended squat while he penetrates her.

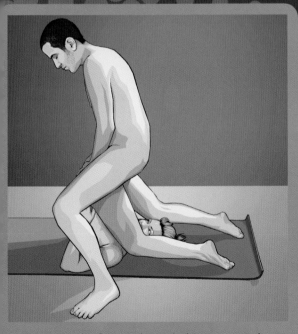

To penetrate her from another angle, he can try reversing his pile-driving stance by facing away from her.

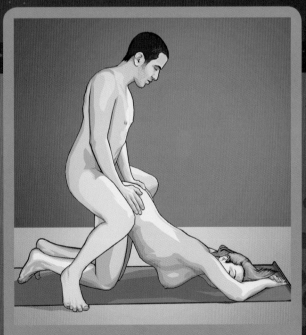

In this less-challenging modification, she kneels, with her behind as high in the air as possible, and he stands over her.

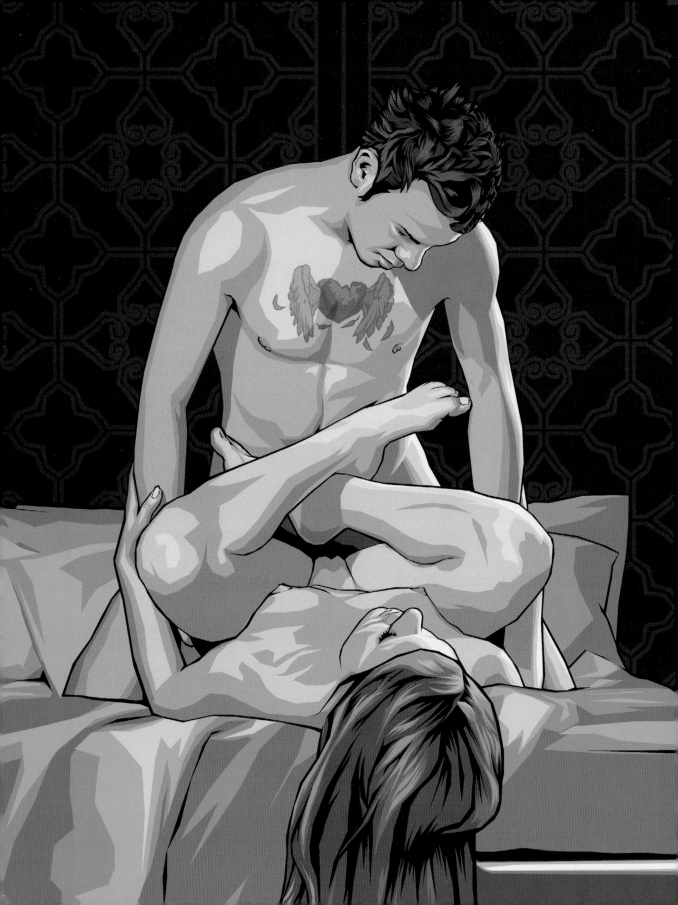

A little variation may bring a lot of pleasure. For instance, a cross-legged version of the missionary position offers sexy views and an interesting angle.

MISSIONARY WITH A TWIST 67

The key to keeping any position fresh is variety—small adjustments can make a world of difference, and being open to trying a range of things can help you find those unexpected variations that drive you wild. There's an infinite range of positions out there. So once you find ones you like, you can start finding ways to make them even more exciting.

For example, during missionary, the woman can bend her knees, twist her knees to the side, wrap her legs around the man's waist, or even cross them.

What can be lovely about this position is its ability to provide a sort of intimate distance—her crossed legs keep him up on his hands, gazing down, rather than pressed close body to body.

Once your bodies are in position, the motion has more to do with rocking and rhythm than hard thrusting. She may want to try lifting her pelvis, perhaps with a pillow under her hips. If her legs get cramped, she can always bring them up and rest them on his shoulders or press her feet against his chest.

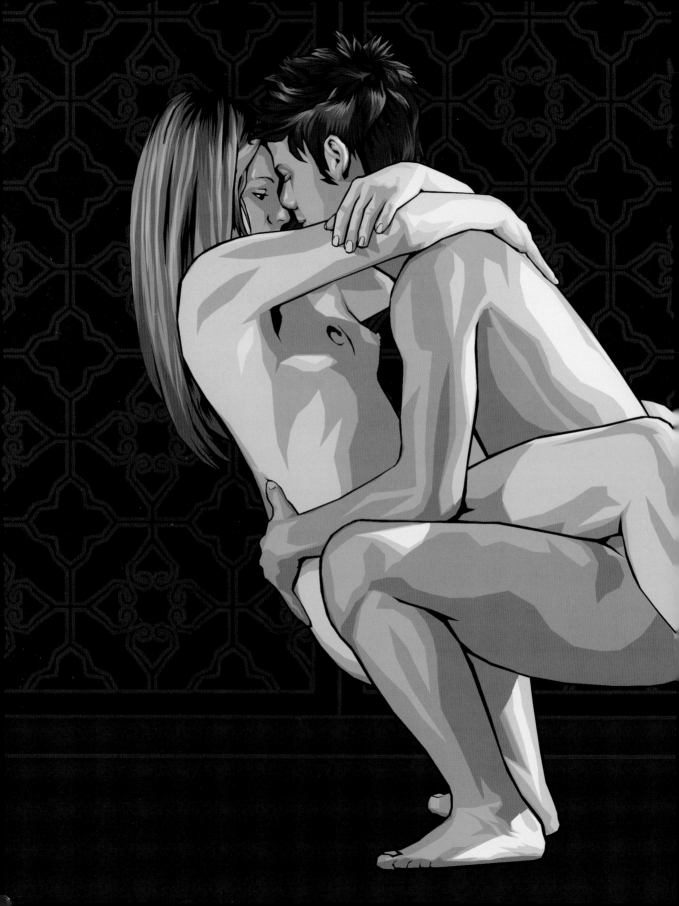

CROUCHING DRAGON

If you've got a healthy back and the legs and upper-arm strength to support your partner, you might want to try out this more advanced sitting position. In lieu of a chair, you use your body to hold her up and keep her close.

To get into the crouching dragon, start by standing up and facing each other. Ask her to wrap her limbs around you: her arms around your neck and her legs around yours. Then squat down while she lowers her body in tandem with yours. Once you're at a level that feels good, ask her to place her thighs, one at a time, over yours. To help you balance, she can press close to you as she grinds onto you; or if you're feeling strong in the stance, she can lean back and thrust from there. After a little bit of time enjoying this position, you can ease forward onto your knees and lower her onto her back for a more conventional man-on-top finish to this athletic endeavor.

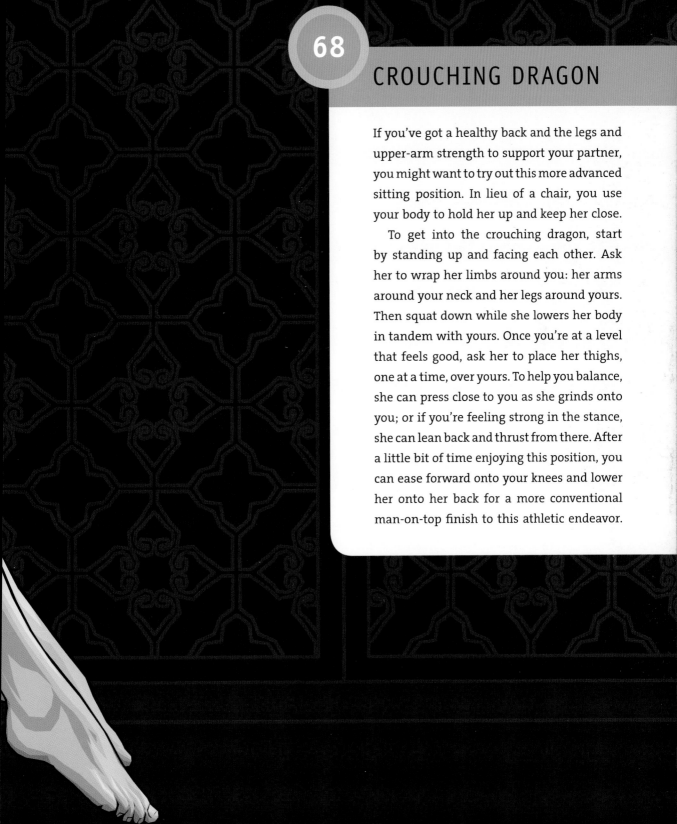

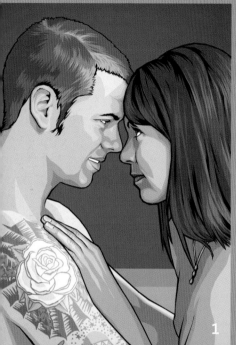

1

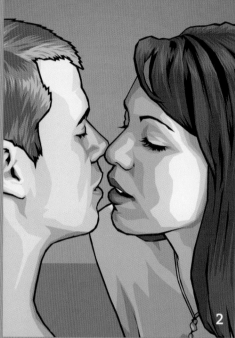

2

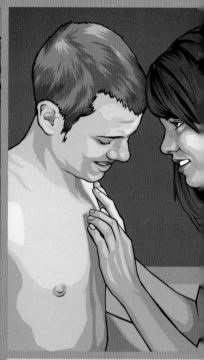

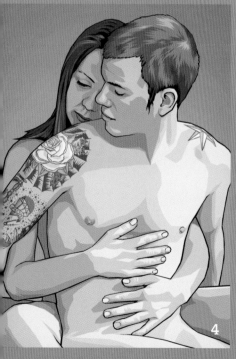

4

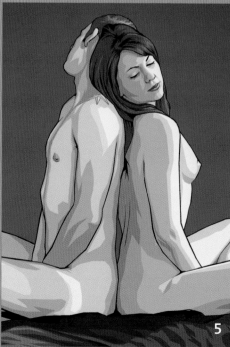

5

{1} Start off by lovingly gazing into each others' nondominant eye (e.g., the left eye for right-handed people). Get close for sensual bond-building.

{2} Gentle kisses awaken desires.

{3} Tapping lightly on your partner's chest and midsection will awaken the heart chakra.

{4} Take turns sitting back to front and using your hands to caress and explore each other.

{5} Sit spine to spine to align your chakras (centers of energy) and sexual electricities.

{6} Yab yum, pictured here, is the traditional tantric position—it can lead to a powerful, explosive finale.

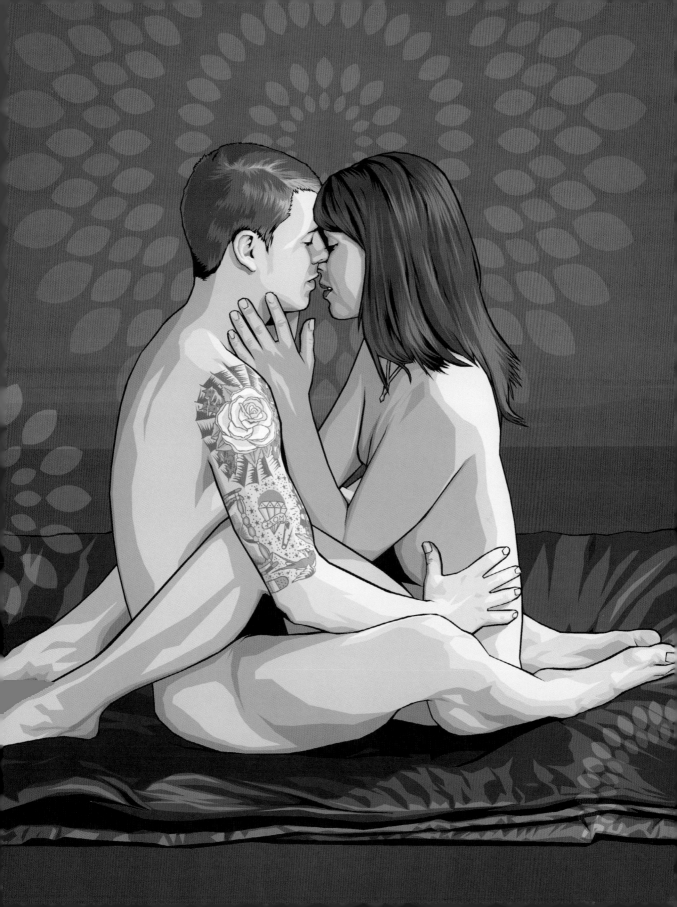

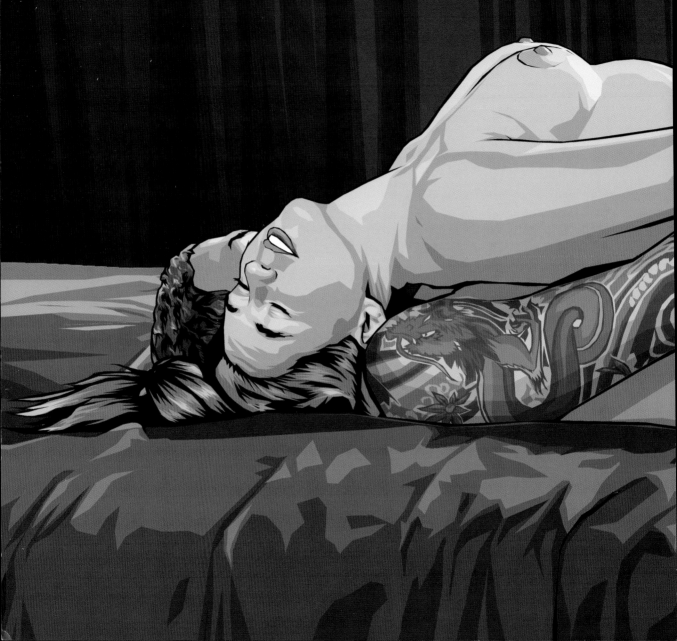

LANGUID BUT LUSTY

In this tantric variation of reverse cowgirl, he's got his knees over the bed, and she's leaning all the way onto his body. This move is great for G-spot stimulation and allows for easy access to her clitoris. He can caress her breasts and kiss her neck while she guides his hands to all the right places, showing him exactly how she likes to be pleasured.

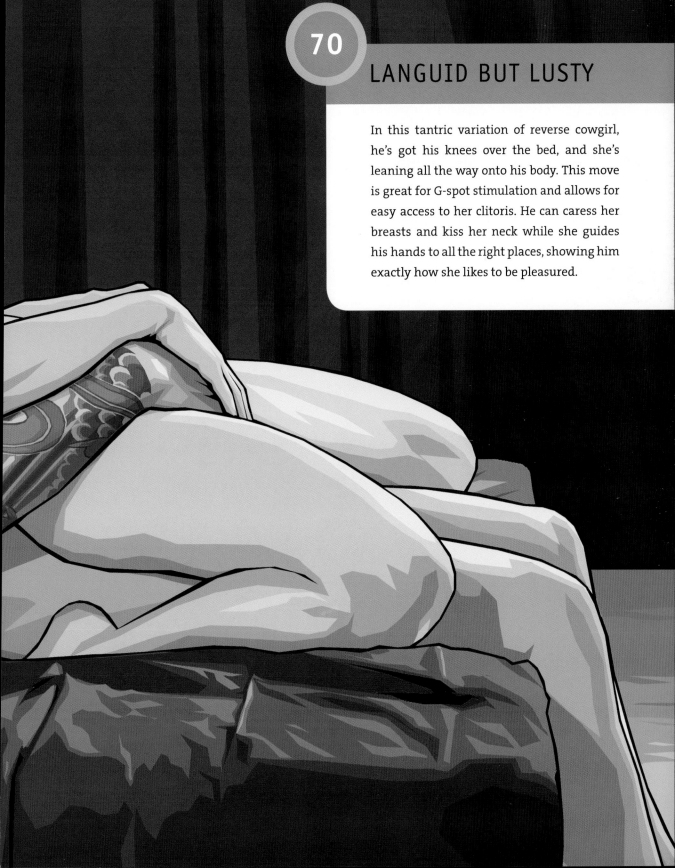

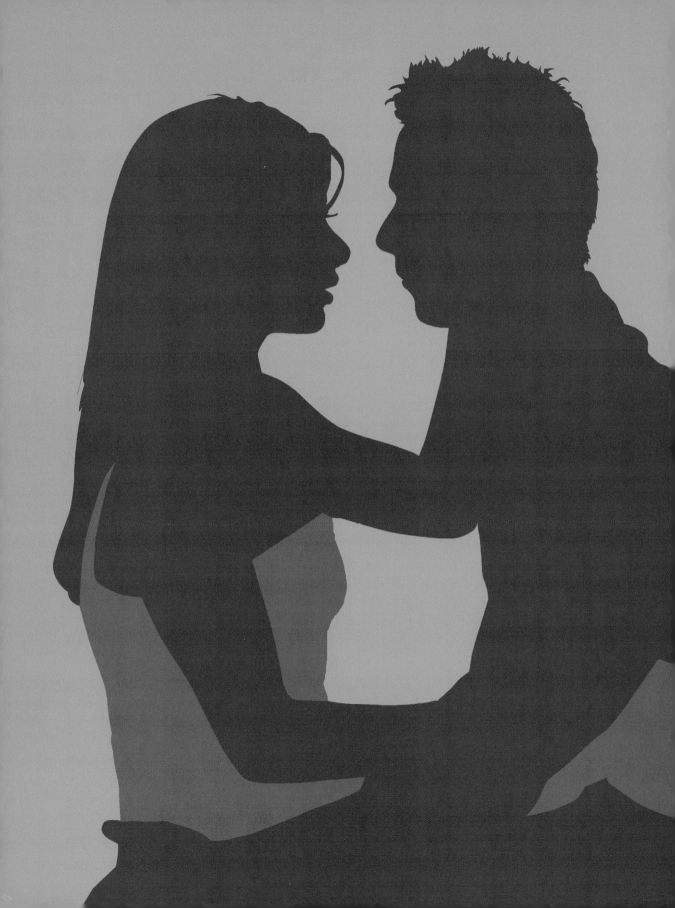

Emily

"**It's quite remarkable** how many couples never talk about sex, yet, communication is essential throughout the cycle—from foreplay to afterglow and everywhere in between. Think about your sex life. Are you and your partner(s) on the same page? Does sex still feel exciting? Engaged? Do you prefer it a little to the left, right, or sideways? No need to rush into new territories, just take your time and talk. Trust builds through shared experiences and through communication. Venture slowly outside your comfort zones to intensify your connection and enhance your relationship as both lovers and friends."

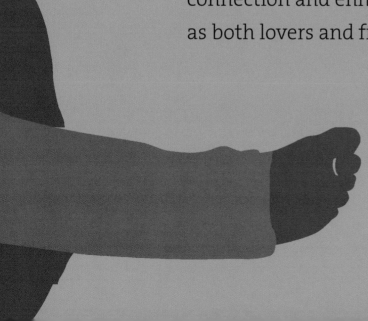

If you're curious about deep throating but anxious about gagging, don't worry. If you wind up telling him that he's too much for you, he'll just be flattered.

71 GOING DOWN—DEEP DOWN

To ease into oral sex, start when he's not erect. Or stick your tongue out to guide him in gently. Not only does this cover your bottom teeth, it also helps you take more of him in. You can also use one or two hands on his shaft and only go down with your mouth as far as it feels comfortable. As long as you keep your hands lubricated with saliva and gently but firmly work the base of his shaft, the sensation will be great for him.

If you want to try taking in more of his penis, focus on your breathing to relax and experiment with different positions to get the alignment exactly right. The variation shown here helps a woman go deeper, because her throat opens up as she leans her head over the bed, and her mouth and throat make a straight line.

Since men come in many shapes, sizes, and curves, it might take a few tries to figure out which position best lines up your throat and his penis. And don't worry about making a bit of noise—men generally relish the sounds women make when they perform oral sex.

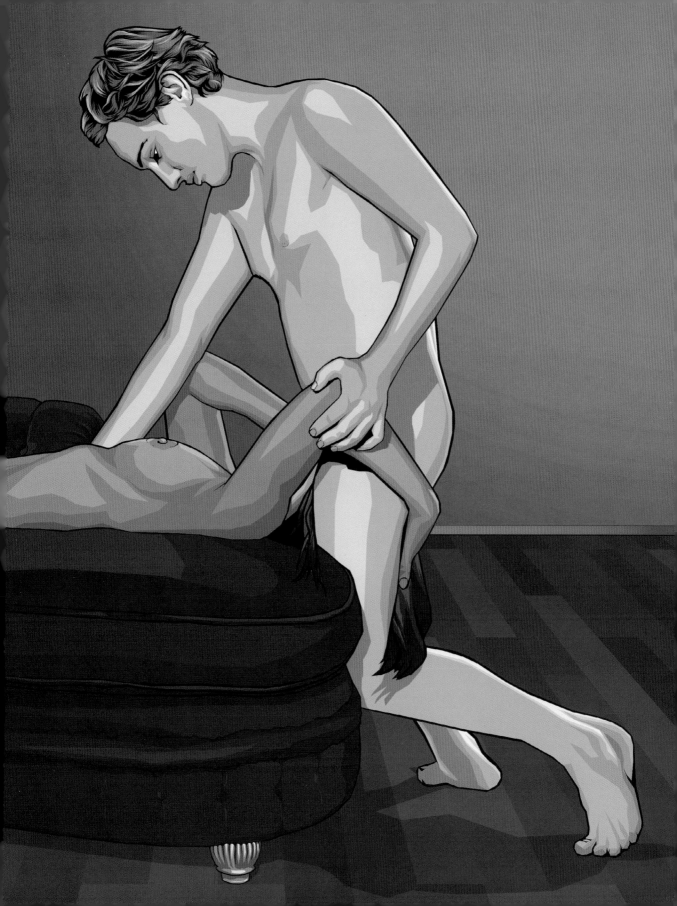

DEEP-THROAT TACTICS

Of course, the dream is to get him all the way down your throat. But give yourself time to build up to this feat: take a little more into the back of your mouth each time—it'll only get easier, and you know he won't complain. You might want to try practicing on a small dildo, or while brushing your teeth (to do this, brush a little farther back on your tongue each time) to master your gag reflex on your own.

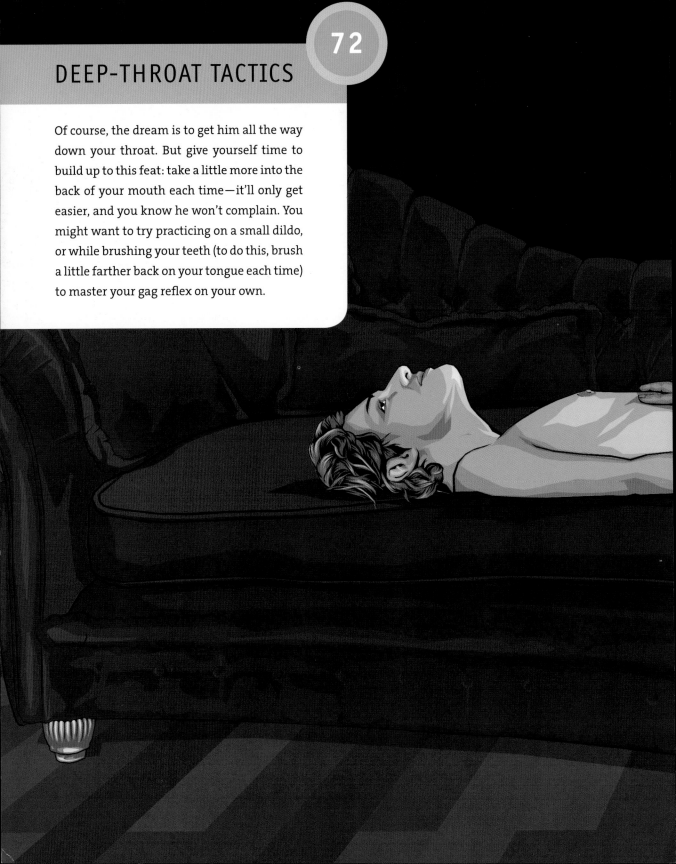

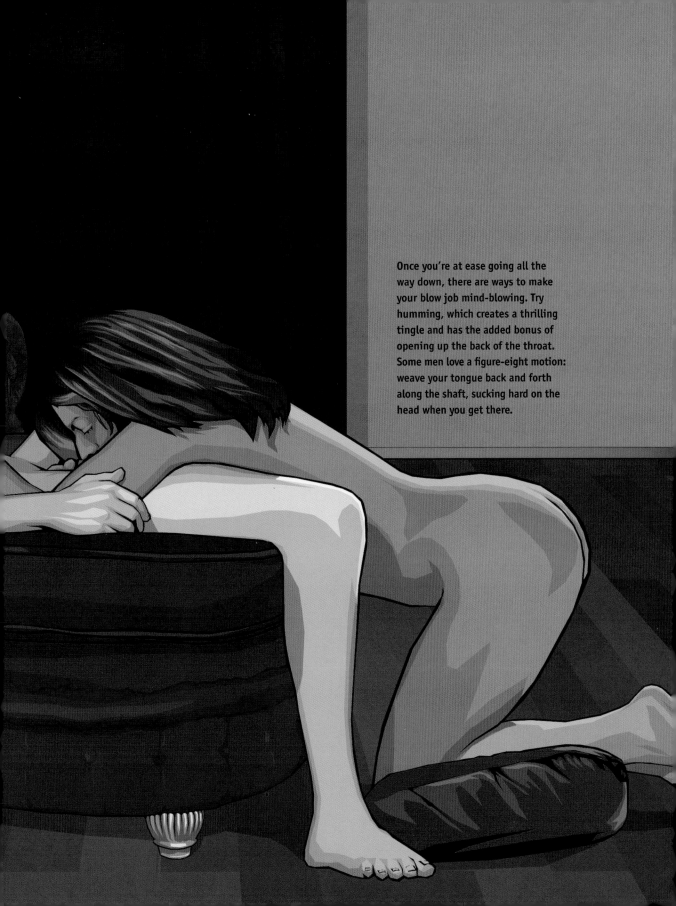

Once you're at ease going all the
way down, there are ways to make
your blow job mind-blowing. Try
humming, which creates a thrilling
tingle and has the added bonus of
opening up the back of the throat.
Some men love a figure-eight motion:
weave your tongue back and forth
along the shaft, sucking hard on the
head when you get there.

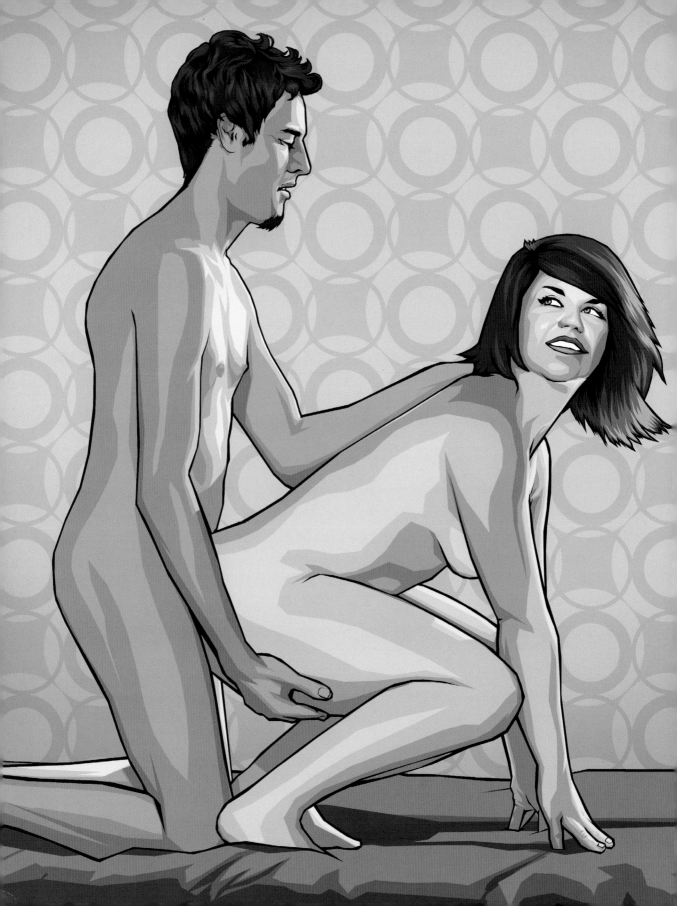

Anal sex can feel good for a number of different reasons—it may stimulate a woman's G-spot, the internal part of her clitoris, or simply her imagination.

BE HER BACKDOOR MAN 73

You might begin anal exploration with a finger, a small dildo, or by putting just the tip of your penis inside her. Ask her to tell you what feels good and what doesn't. Stop if she experiences any pain. Go slowly, and give her a chance to relax and breathe before you go farther in. Positions like doggie-style, missionary, and spooning are likely going to be the easiest for anal intercourse, but you can carefully experiment with many other positions. Use lots of lubrication; silicone- and water-based lubes are most condom-compatible. A concern for a lot of people is cleanliness, but your body is naturally adept at keeping itself clean. If you're in good health, your digestive system is not likely to cause you any problems. (Just be careful not to switch back and forth between vaginal and anal intercourse or even let lube drip from one place to the other.) Using condoms adds insurance—and is crucial for safer sex.

Some couples enjoy anal sex regularly; others like it every now and again. Give it a try and if you don't like it, move on.

EXPLORING ALTERNATIVES

There are many sensitive nerve endings right around the entrance of the anus, so you can pleasure your partner with light touching or licking. If you choose to probe deeper, the basic guidelines are the same as for anal intercourse: relax, breathe, talk, and lubricate. Both the prostate and the internal part of the clitoris can be stimulated through anal play. Start out slowly and stop when necessary. This simple formula can help you get comfortable enough to climax.

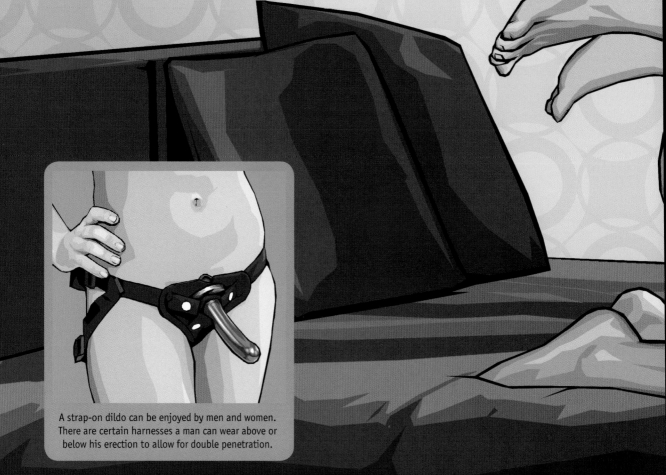

A strap-on dildo can be enjoyed by men and women. There are certain harnesses a man can wear above or below his erection to allow for double penetration.

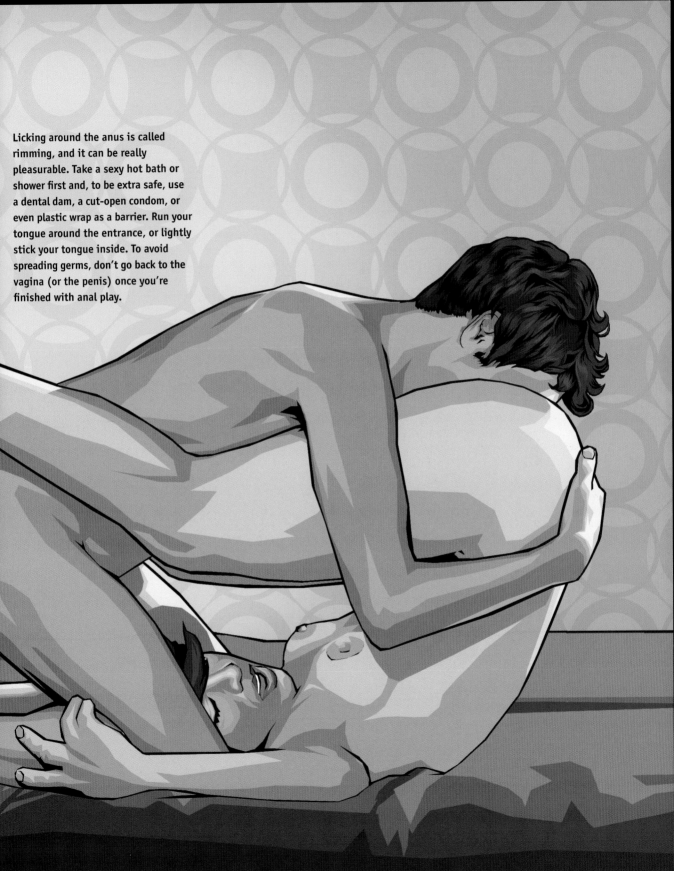

Licking around the anus is called rimming, and it can be really pleasurable. Take a sexy hot bath or shower first and, to be extra safe, use a dental dam, a cut-open condom, or even plastic wrap as a barrier. Run your tongue around the entrance, or lightly stick your tongue inside. To avoid spreading germs, don't go back to the vagina (or the penis) once you're finished with anal play.

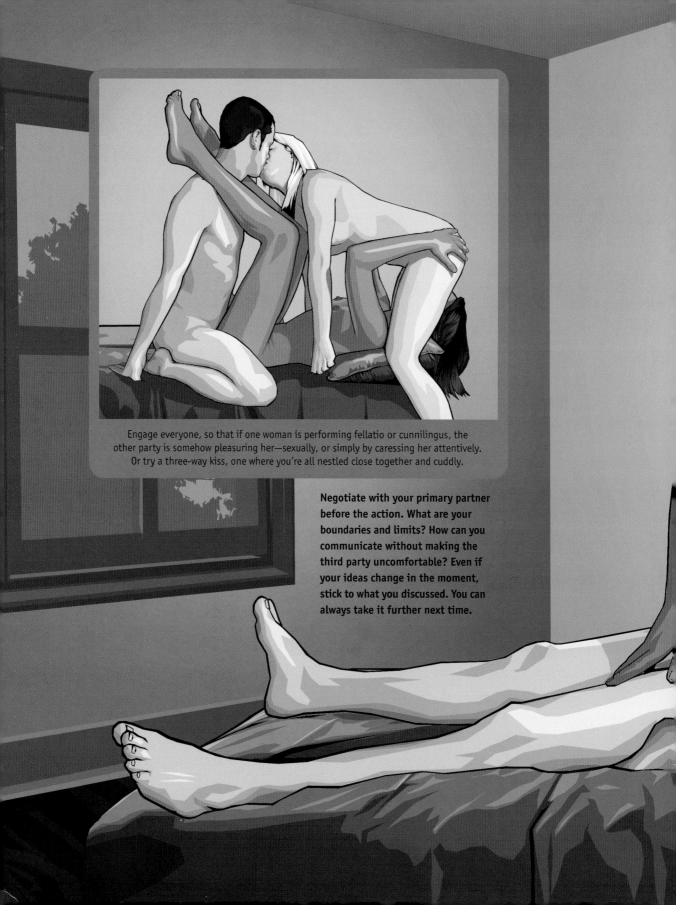

Engage everyone, so that if one woman is performing fellatio or cunnilingus, the other party is somehow pleasuring her—sexually, or simply by caressing her attentively. Or try a three-way kiss, one where you're all nestled close together and cuddly.

Negotiate with your primary partner before the action. What are your boundaries and limits? How can you communicate without making the third party uncomfortable? Even if your ideas change in the moment, stick to what you discussed. You can always take it further next time.

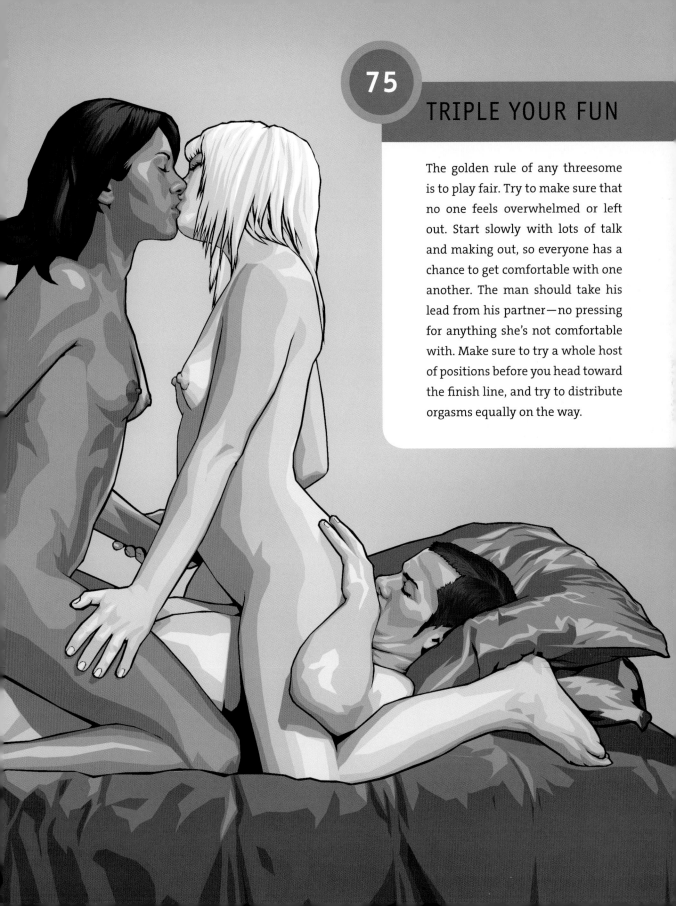

75

TRIPLE YOUR FUN

The golden rule of any threesome is to play fair. Try to make sure that no one feels overwhelmed or left out. Start slowly with lots of talk and making out, so everyone has a chance to get comfortable with one another. The man should take his lead from his partner—no pressing for anything she's not comfortable with. Make sure to try a whole host of positions before you head toward the finish line, and try to distribute orgasms equally on the way.

Threesomes with two women are more common, but don't forget that ladies enjoy being the center of attention as well, and men can make it happen.

76 SHARING THE MOMENT

It's a simple fact that women tend to be more comfortable than men about being physical together. This doesn't rule out the possibility of a great man-woman-man threesome—but you may need a little more negotiation and discussion with all parties before the action begins.

Some men are really into the fantasy of sharing a woman, but don't want to touch each other at all. All that means for the woman is that she's going to have even more attention lavished on her, since the men won't be playing together.

If the men are comfortable with more contact, and if the woman is interested in being adventurous, they may wish to try double penetration. She gets on top of one partner and leans forward, pressing her chest into his, while the second man enters her anally from behind.

As with any group adventure, make sure that everyone agrees on the ground rules before any clothes come off, always practice safe sex, and take care that you pay lots of attention to your primary partner to avoid any jealousy.

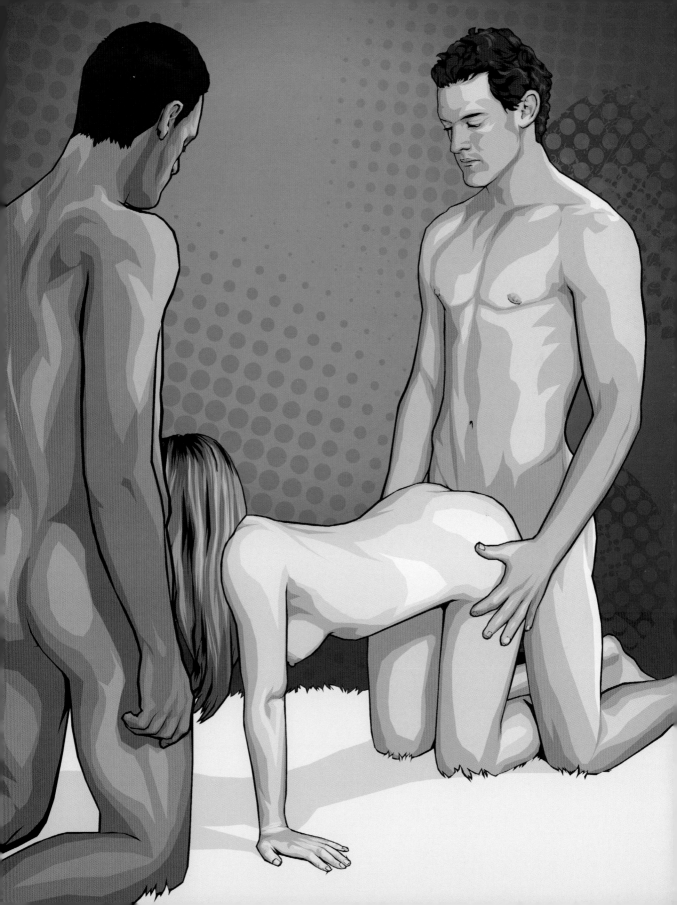

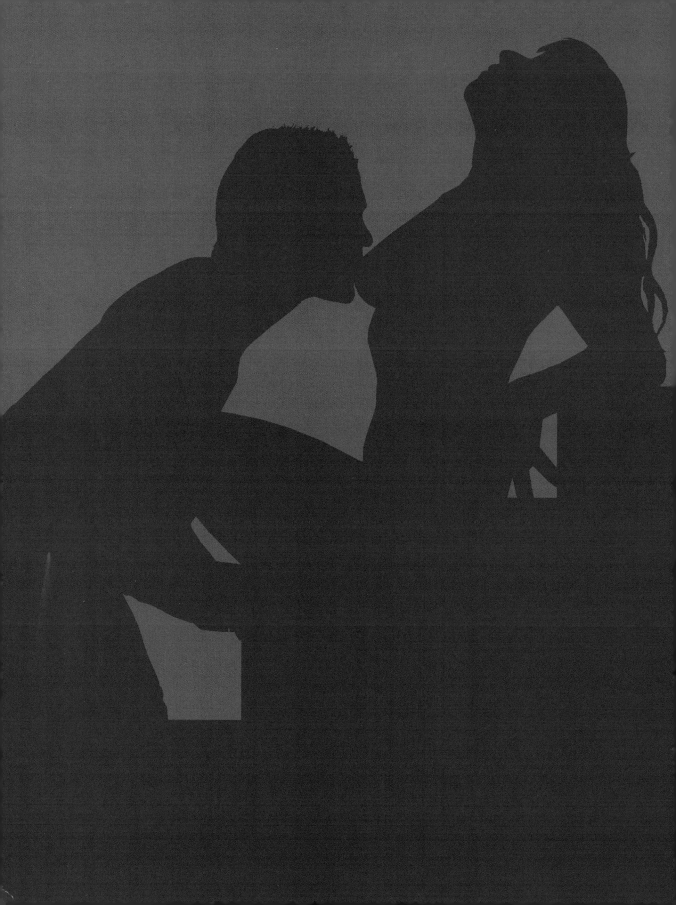

Emily

"**The chance of** getting caught fuels the passion—plus there's nothing like getting away with it. Sex in nature is always a fun addition to outdoor activities. Tuck yourselves away from others in the bushes or on hidden paths to experience the thrill and enchantment of the outdoors."

Jamye

"**Some of the hottest** places I've had sex include a bench next to the track at my college and the stairwell in an office building. A hand job under a blanket in an airplane was also unforgettable. Adventurous locations make for lifelong memories, so grab them when you can."

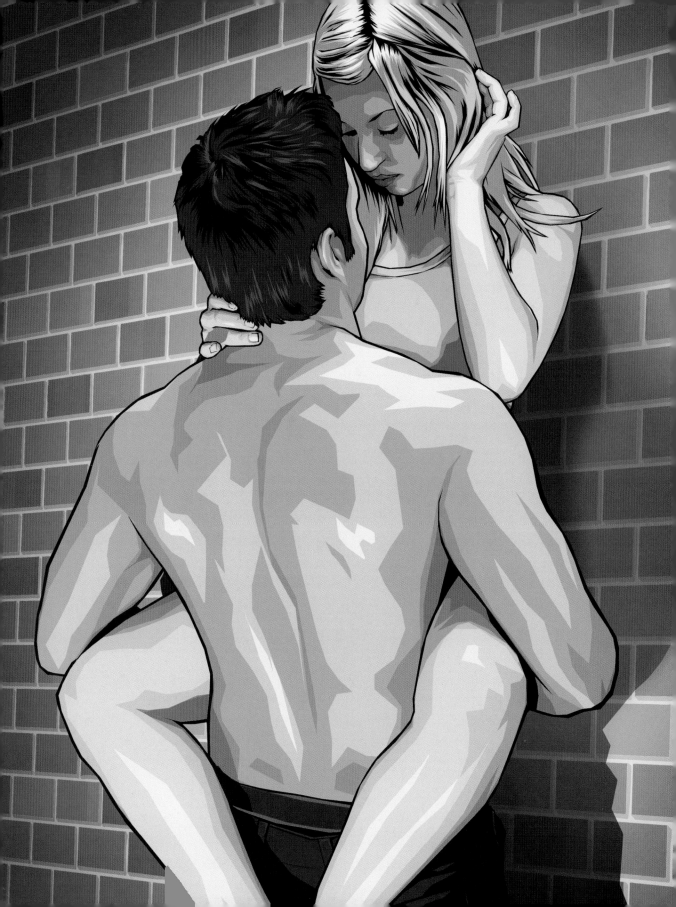

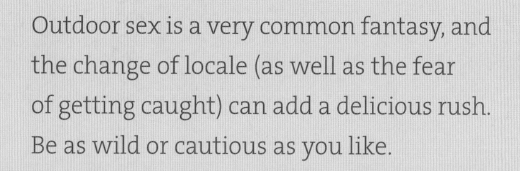

Outdoor sex is a very common fantasy, and the change of locale (as well as the fear of getting caught) can add a delicious rush. Be as wild or cautious as you like.

Use some discretion as you plan your al fresco exploits. After all, outdoor sex is generally not legal and certainly not appreciated by most passersby. If you're worried about getting caught, you can experience a bit of the thrill by fooling around on your apartment's balcony, or in your backyard, a garage, or a pool. (Just make sure the fence is high enough that your neighbors don't get a free show).

From there, you can work your way up to racier spots. The woman should wear a skirt with no panties, and guys need pants that unzip so it's easy for you to make a quick and at least semiclothed getaway in case you have to make a mad dash for it. Make sure you choose a safe area, and watch out for cameras or other security devices. You don't want to trip someone's motion-detecting alarm.

Scouting for sexotic venues? L'amour at the beach is a good choice, because you're weightless in water, which also provides the perfect cover for friskier activities. Or try something grittier, like a public restroom in your favorite club.

Sneaking into your office to have a quickie with your partner can be a lot of fun—and afterward, you'll smile every time you sit down at your desk.

78 PUTTING IN SOME OVERTIME

Go in after hours, on weekends, or early in the morning, before your coworkers are there. Find out where the security cameras are so that you don't get caught on tape. If you want to be ultraprepared, bring a bag of gym clothes to work with you. This way you can always say you came up to the office to change before or after a workout, a plausible excuse regardless of the hour.

Plan carefully, noting your colleagues' schedules, especially those who work long hours or on weekends. Then stake out a place or two to make it happen. Perhaps your cubicle is hidden in the corner, or you have your own private office, or you know of a closet that locks. The perfect spot for some office nookie may be the bathroom, since it's illegal to put cameras there. So lock the door, or hang up an "out of order" sign. No matter how spicy it sounds, doing the deed during regular office hours is not the best idea. It's far wiser to wait for the off-hours, or find somewhere that you're confident is really secret and secure.

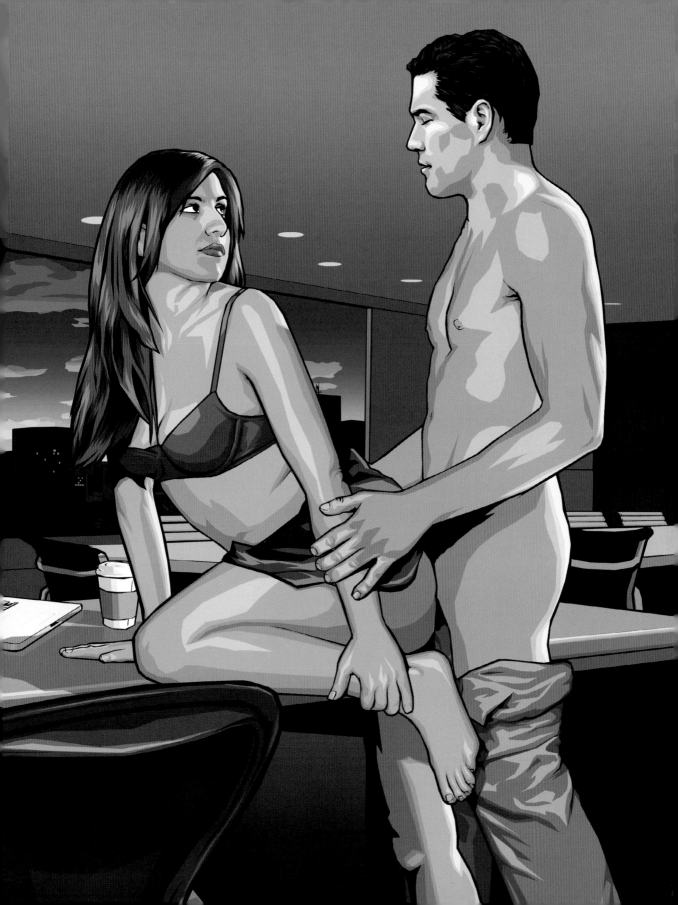

GETTING OFF THE BEATEN TRACK

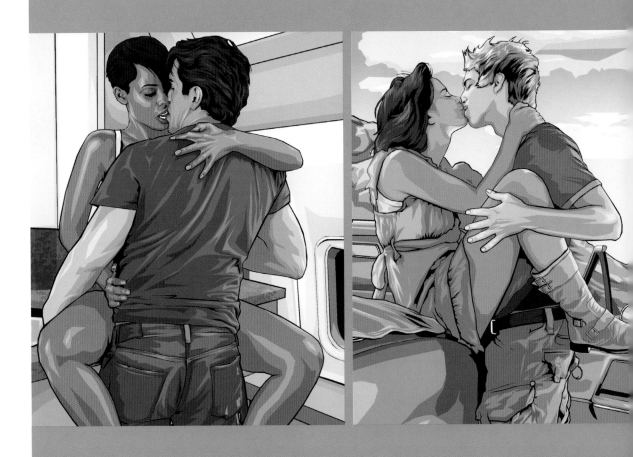

MILE-HIGH CLUB This is easiest on a long flight, especially an overnighter. Sneak into the bathroom together, or if you're the only two in your row, grab blankets and get it on once the captain has turned off the seatbelt sign.

ON THE HOOD Doing it on the hood of your car is a far less cramped experience than a traditional backseat encounter. Choose somewhere safe and secluded, and put a blanket (or a jacket) between you and the paint job for comfort.

SEX IN EXOTIC SPOTS IS THE KIND THAT EARNS YOU BRAGGING RIGHTS.

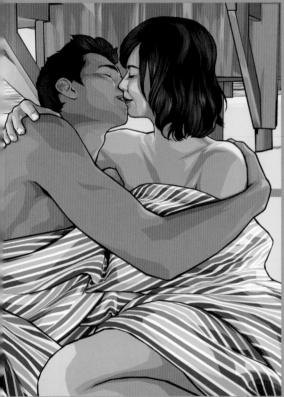

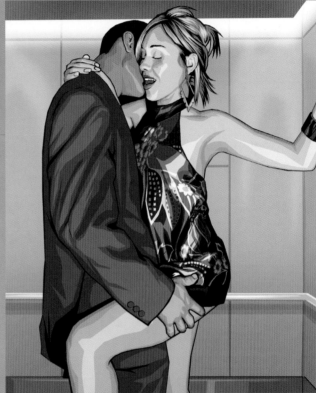

UNDER THE BOARDWALK There's a lot that's erotic about the beach—you're likely relaxed, scantily clad, slathered in lotion, and warmed by the sun. When you get down, put a towel over you, and consider keeping the bikini bottoms on.

IN THE ELEVATOR Search for a building with a lot of floors and little activity. Do it in a back corner so that you have a second to adjust yourselves when the doors open. Or hit the emergency stop button to give yourselves more time.

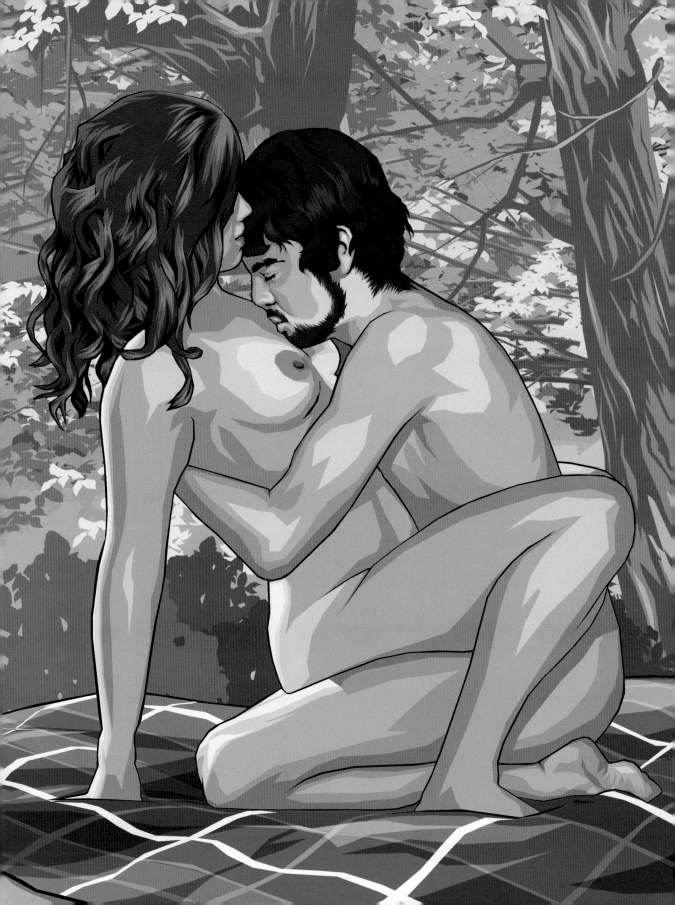

Sex in the great outdoors can be stunningly sensual. Get in touch with your animal instincts, or make up your own fantasy about a modern Garden of Eden.

A NATURAL HIGH 80

You might be overtaken by feelings of passion while out on a hike. Or you might be packing for a full-scale erotic camping trip. Either way, the experience can be enhanced by just a little planning.

If you want to dart off the trail and do it like bunnies, take the time to find a spot that's semiremote, obscured by trees, or behind big rocks. Be sure to avoid any stinging plants or thorny bushes.

For a less impromptu frolic, set up a rustic but romantic campsite, complete with a comfortable air mattress in your tent. Remember that just because no one can see you in your tent doesn't mean they can't hear you. Keep quiet if you want to avoid startling park rangers, other campers, and, of course, the animals.

Finally, make sure to clean up after yourselves. Wash up in a lake, stream, or waterfall, and remove all evidence of your excursion—including condoms, wrappers, sex toys, and anything else you brought along to the woods or mountains. You'll still have your memories, and Mother Nature doesn't need souvenirs.

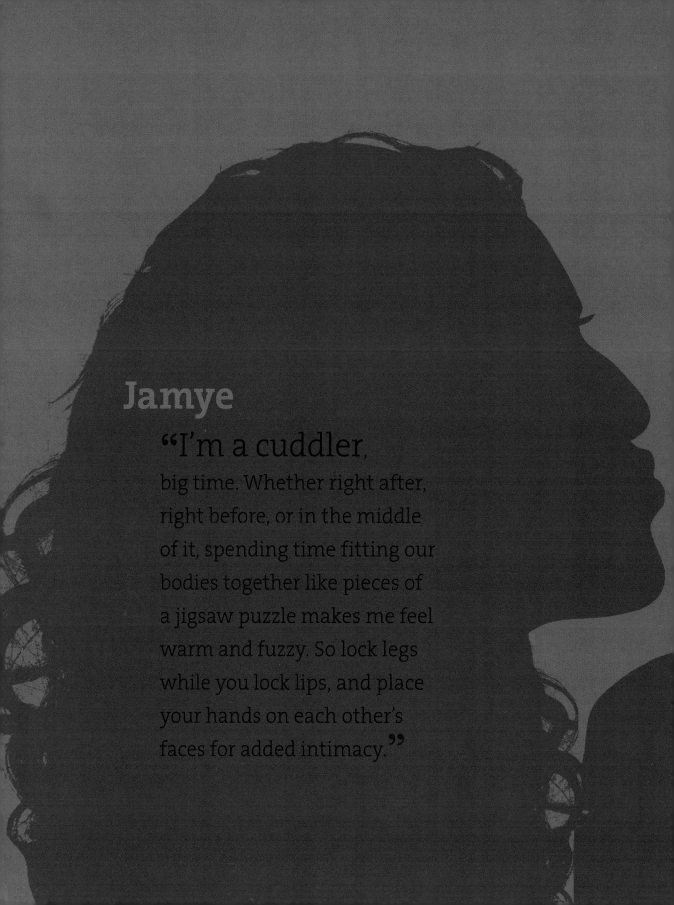

Jamye

"I'm a cuddler, big time. Whether right after, right before, or in the middle of it, spending time fitting our bodies together like pieces of a jigsaw puzzle makes me feel warm and fuzzy. So lock legs while you lock lips, and place your hands on each other's faces for added intimacy."

Emily

"Ah, the postcoital glow. After you go to the bathroom (it's important for women to empty their bladders after lovemaking), it's time to settle in for some cuddling. Plus, oxytocin (the cuddle hormone) spikes in both men and women during sex and primes us for some serious bonding time."

Sex in a hot tub or spa is a common fantasy that can make for a mind-blowing reality. Before you take the plunge, there are a few little things you should know.

81 GETTING INTO HOT WATER

The very first thing you might want to consider is what's in the water besides the two of you. If enjoying your own hot tub, be sure you use the least irritating cleaning products possible. In a public tub, the water probably contains a lot of chlorine or other chemicals—you may want to avoid them if you're sensitive.

When you're ready to get wet and wild, have lots of silicone lube on hand. Sex in water washes away a woman's natural lubrication, but silicone lube has staying power. Then pick the position that captures your fancy. The woman can hold on to the side while the man enters her from behind, or he can sit on one of the benches with the woman astride him, either facing him or facing away. Don't forget to incorporate the water jets into the fun. Many women find them a fantastic way to have an orgasm.

When your session's over, you should both be sure to get out of the tub and pee. It's a good idea to go to the bathroom before and after sex, to prevent infections, and after hot-tub sex it's extra important.

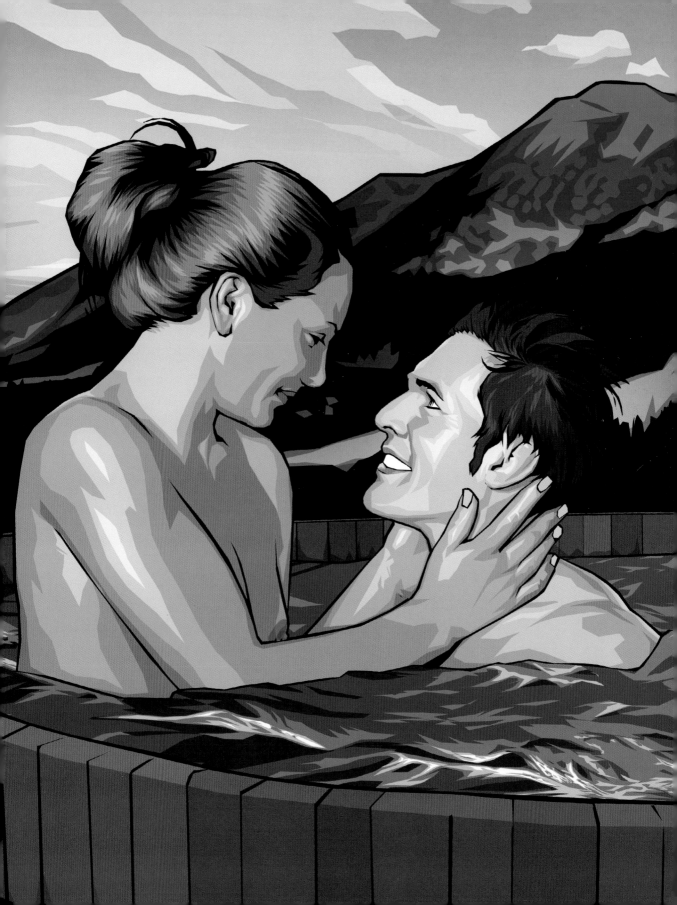

SHOWERED WITH LOVE

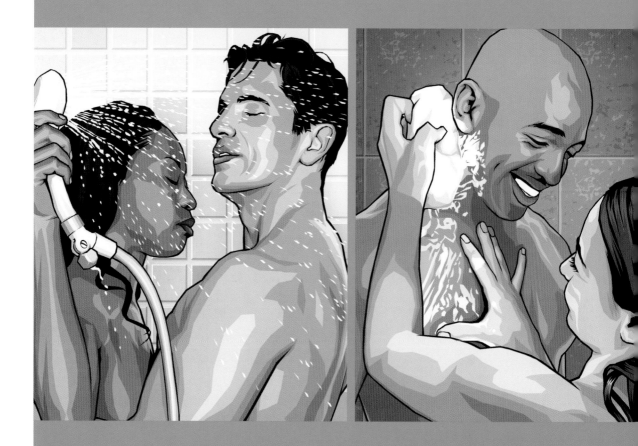

SHOWER SEX-CESSORIES A sponge, a washcloth, or a handheld shower nozzle can all be sex toys. Gently loofah the inner thighs or direct a spray of water right on those sensitive areas. A double-headed shower is the dream, of course.

KEEP IT CLEAN Washing your partner's privates is an obvious move, but don't lose sight of how sensual it is to wash and suds down your lover's entire body. Grab a soapy sponge and circle it over everything *but* those hot spots.

GETTING DIRTY IS FUN—AND SO IS GETTING CLEAN, IF YOU DO IT RIGHT.

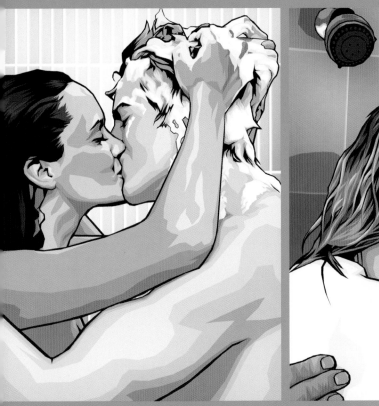

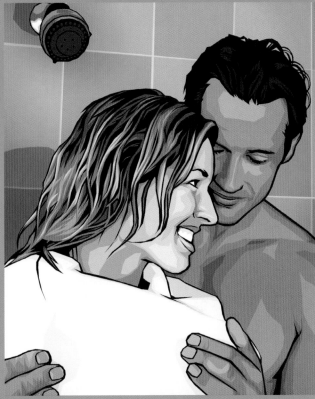

SENSUAL SHAMPOO A scalp massage can relax and revive the entire body. Lather up with shampoo, then start at the base of the neck and rub the pads of your fingers in a circular motion. Up the pressure, and continue all over the head.

STAY IN THE MOMENT After a steamy shower, don't just hop out and dry off. Keep the connection going by staying in the steam and drying each other off— slowly, gently, and ever-so-thoroughly. This may lead you into round two.

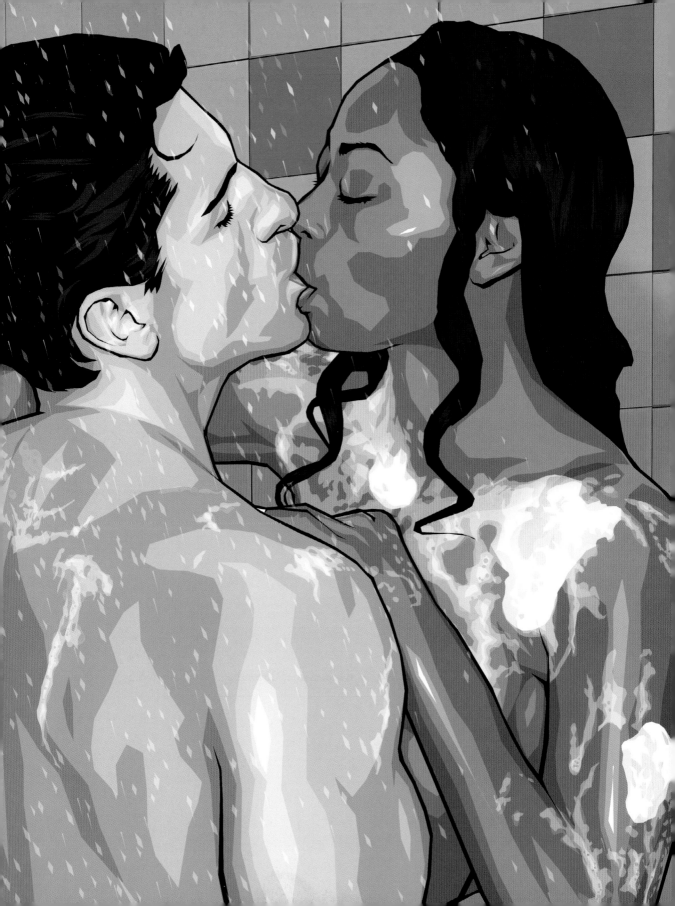

Don't stop when you've had enough. Make good vibrations last by cuddling with your partner and tuning in to each other so you both know how special your bond is.

NEVER STOP EXPLORING (83)

Whether it was hot and fast, slow and sensual, or all of the above, sex isn't over when it stops. So take care of both yourself and your partner when you're done with the heat of the moment. Savor those most recent sensations, as well as your ongoing connection. You can stay in bed and snooze for another five minutes before preparing for your day or watch a movie and cuddle on the couch. Whatever you choose to do, try to spend at least a little time reconnecting before you peel your bodies apart.

If you have to run off instead of enjoying the afterglow, be sure to send a text or call during the day. Talk about how you felt and how much fun you had. Right before you go to sleep, let your partner know that you love being together.

Love isn't only about sex. Love is a decision, and it requires preparation and work. It goes beyond the bedroom. Even if you have to schedule sex, when it's time to be with the person who turns you on, stay tuned in. That's the greatest gift of all—for your partner and for you.

GLOSSARY OF ANATOMICAL TERMS

EXTERNAL FEMALE ORGANS

INTERNAL FEMALE ORGANS

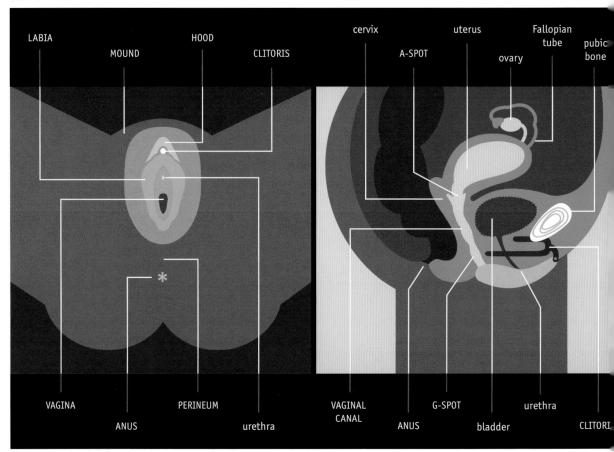

A-SPOT The anterior fornix spot, an erogenous zone located above the G-spot, near the cervix.

ANUS The opening to the rectum, located between the buttocks.

AREOLA The colored ring around the nipple.

CLITORIS The organ primarily responsible for female orgasm. Only a small portion of the clitoris is visible—most of it exists internally.

FORESKIN Loose skin that protects the head of a man's penis. The foreskin itself is quite sensitive for many men.

FRENULUM A sensitive spot just below the head of the penis, which faces away from the body when the penis is erect.

G-SPOT The Grafenberg spot, an erogenous zone located on the front wall of the vagina.

HEAD (GLANS) The tip of the penis. Also slang for oral sex.

HOOD The piece of skin that protects the clitoris. It is quite sensitive in and of itself for many women.

LABIA The vaginal lips, consisting of the outer lips (labia majora)—which form the outer limits of the female genitalia—and the inner lips (labia minora), which run from the clitoral hood to below the vaginal opening.

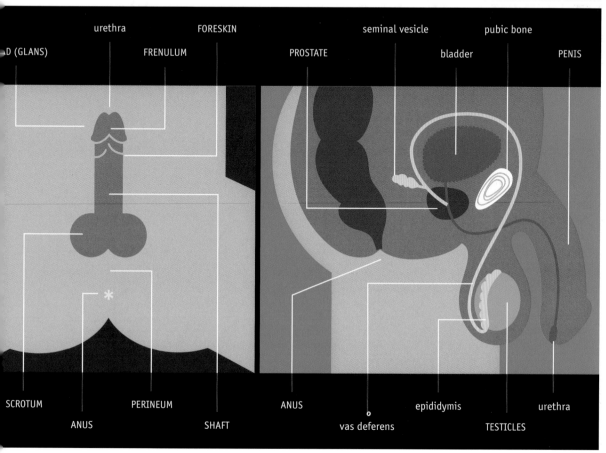

urethra
FORESKIN
seminal vesicle
pubic bone

D (GLANS)
FRENULUM
PROSTATE
bladder
PENIS

*

SCROTUM
ANUS
PERINEUM
SHAFT
ANUS
vas deferens
epididymis
TESTICLES
urethra

MOUND Fleshy spot right above a woman's genital area.

PELVIC FLOOR MUSCLES The muscles connecting and supporting most of the sexual organs, bladder, anus, etc.

PENIS The male sexual organ.

PERINEUM The area between the sexual organs and the anus.

PROSTATE The gland responsible for some of the fluid in male ejaculate. Can be a source of sexual pleasure.

PUBOCOCCYGEUS (PC) MUSCLE The muscle exercised in Kegels, found in both genders (see General Glossary).

RECTUM The passage just inside the anus.

SCROTUM The external pouch that contains a man's testicles.

SHAFT The main body of the penis, exclusive of the head. In general, term is used only to refer to the erect organ.

TESTICLES The glands that produce sperm; often called "balls."

VAGINA Technically, the vaginal canal. The term "vagina" is often incorrectly used to refer to all of a woman's sexual organs.

VAGINAL CANAL Passage connecting the vaginal opening to the uterus.

VULVA The entire external female genital area. The term "vagina" is often mistakenly used as a synonym.

GENERAL GLOSSARY

ANAL SEX Penetration of the anus for sexual purposes.

BDSM Abbreviation for bondage/discipline + dominance/submission + sadism/masochism. BDSM play may involve any or all of these practices.

BLOW JOB See *Fellatio*.

BONDAGE Physical restraint often used in sexual play.

BOTTOM The "receiver" of a sexual act. Usually, but not exclusively, used in a BDSM context.

CHAKRA One of seven "energy points" that exist on the human body according to tantric practice.

CIRCUMCISION An operation that removes most of the foreskin of the penis. Female circumcision also exists; it is widely considered to be a form of genital mutilation.

COITAL ALIGNMENT TECHNIQUE (CAT) A sexual position in which the man positions himself so as to directly stimulate the clitoris with the shaft of his penis.

CONDOM A sheath, often of latex, made to cover the penis; used for birth control and disease prevention. The female condom is a larger sheath that can be used to line the vagina or rectum for similar protection.

COWGIRL Sexual position in which the woman straddles the man, face to face. When she faces his feet, it's called "reverse cowgirl."

CROCODILE CLAMPS Adjustable nipple clamps with metal teeth, usually cushioned with soft rubber.

CUNNILINGUS Oral sex on a woman.

DEEP THROAT Fellatio in which the man's penis, or a dildo, is taken entirely into the mouth and throat.

DENTAL DAM A thin square of latex designed for dental work; used for safer oral sex and rimming.

DILDO A nonvibrating toy designed for vaginal or anal insertion. Dildos can be penis-shaped or take other forms, and be made of stainless steel, silicone, glass, or a range of other materials.

DISCIPLINE The consensual practice of "punishment" in a sexual context.

DOGGIE STYLE Sexual position with the woman on her knees and the man kneeling behind her.

DOMINANCE The act of taking control in a sexual context.

DOUBLE PENETRATION Sex act in which a woman experiences simultaneous penetration of both the vagina and anus.

EJACULATE The fluid (usually) released from a man's penis at orgasm; the act of emitting said fluid. See also *Female Ejaculation*.

ENDORPHINS Neurotransmitters that perform a wide range of functions, including being responsible for the "high" felt as the result of intense stimulation.

EROGENOUS ZONE Any area of the human body that experiences heightened sensitivity when stimulated. These zones vary widely from person to person.

FEMALE EJACULATION The emission of fluid from around a woman's urethra during orgasm. While the fluid is not believed to be urine, its exact makeup is the subject of much debate. Also called "squirting."

FANTASY Mental imagery that is sexually stimulating.

FELLATIO Oral sex on a man. The slang term "blow job" is often used.

FLOGGER A toy made of multiple strands of leather or other materials.

FOOTSIE A flirtatious move in which one party rubs the other's feet, legs, or other areas with their foot.

FOREPLAY Any acts leading up to sexual intercourse.

FROTTAGE The sexual act of rubbing against an object or person.

GENITALS The sexual and reproductive organs.

KAMA SUTRA Classical Indian text describing a wide variety of sexual practices.

KEGELS Exercises that involve squeezing and releasing the PC muscle. The best way to find this muscle is, while urinating, to stop the flow momentarily. Then, practice tensing and releasing it at other times.

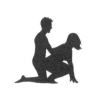   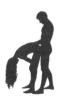

LUBE Lubricant, used for vaginal, anal, and manual sex, as well as for massage. Can be water-, silicone-, or oil-based. Oil-based lubes cannot be used with condoms.

MANUAL An action that involves use of the hands.

MASOCHIST Someone who enjoys feeling consensually agreed-to pain or discomfort in a sexual situation.

MASTURBATE To manually stimulate the genitals. Usually used to indicate self-pleasure.

MILE-HIGH CLUB An imaginary club composed of people who have had sex on an airplane.

MISSIONARY The traditional man-on-top sexual position.

MUTUAL MASTURBATION Sex act in which partners masturbate themselves in close proximity, or masturbate each other.

ORAL Having to do with the mouth.

ORGASM A series of highly pleasurable rhythmic contractions as a result of sexual activity.

PEGGING Anal penetration of a man with a strap-on dildo.

PILE DRIVER An advanced sex position in which the man stands over the woman, who is in an inverted pose.

PLAY Refers to any sort of sexual or sexualized activity (as in "role play") or contact (as in "anal play").

PRIMARY PARTNER The person with whom one intends to have the deepest emotional and sexual bond.

REAR ENTRY Sexual position in which the man enters the woman from behind; can be used to refer to vaginal or anal sex.

RIMMING Sex act involving oral stimulation of the anus.

ROLE PLAY Used when partners take on personas for flirting, sex play, and/or intercourse. May involve elaborate costumes and backstories, or something as simple as one person dominating another.

SADIST An individual who enjoys inflicting consensually agreed-to pain or discomfort in a sexual situation.

SAFE WORD A term used to stop or slow down the action in a sexual situation. The word is negotiated before foreplay and can be used at any time to communicate physical or mental discomfort and end a particular action.

SAFER SEX Sex in which bodily fluids are not exchanged (to avoid pregnancy or infection). Usually refers to condom use for intercourse or oral sex, although also covers oral sex using a dental dam or other barrier method.

SEXERCISE Vigorous, athletic, or physically challenging sex. Also, exercises used to strengthen or stretch muscles in preparation.

SEXTING The act of sending racy or explicit messages or photos via text message.

SILICONE A manmade material used for lubes and sex toys. Silicone toys are nonporous, nontoxic, and top-rack–dishwasher safe. Silicone lube is waterproof and extra slick.

69 Any oral sex position in which partners pleasure each other simultaneously.

STRAP-ON A dildo worn in a harness, for ease of penetration.

SUBMISSION The act of giving up control in a sexual situation.

TANTRA Spiritual sex practices that draw on a variety of Eastern writings about sex and spirituality.

THREESOME A sexual experience involving three people. These are often referred to as "MMF" (two males, one female) or "FFM" (two females, one male).

TOP The active performer, or "giver," of a sexual act. Often, but not exclusively, used in a BDSM context.

TOY Any device used for sexual teasing or pleasure.

TWEEZER CLAMPS Nipple clamps with long, thin adjustable arms.

VIBRATOR Any sex toy that vibrates—may be insertable or not.

YAB YUM Tantric sexual position in which the man and woman sit facing each other.

TOY GALLERY

There are so many toys to choose from. Basic models are made by a wide variety of manufacturers, in a range of colors, shapes, and sizes. Others are highly proprietary and made by only one company. Below, some of the most popular or top-of-the line of every kind—most also have a world of variation to explore that there simply wasn't room to show in this space, so shop around and see what looks good to you.

Finger-mounted vibrator

Available in hard and soft models, these vibes slip conveniently over a finger (yours or a partner's) for hands-on vibrations. (ScreamingO FingO)

VIBRATORS

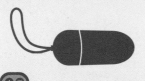

Remote-control egg

This vibrator is inserted, and then turned on, up, or off by a remote control. Other models exist without the remote, but this option is a lot of fun in public.

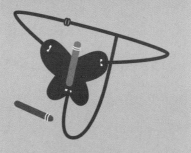

Wearable vibrator

Designed to fit right over the clitoris and under clothes, this device can be worn anywhere. Except maybe the pool.

Waterproof mini vibe

Small "pocket rocket" designed to fit discreetly into a purse and go everywhere, including the shower. (Vibratex Water Dancer)

Palm vibrator

A vibrator curved to perfectly fit the hand and simultaneously stimulate both the clitoris and vaginal lips. (LELO Nea)

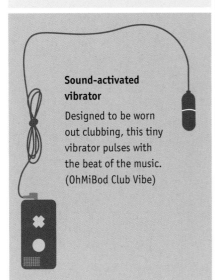

Sound-activated vibrator

Designed to be worn out clubbing, this tiny vibrator pulses with the beat of the music. (OhMiBod Club Vibe)

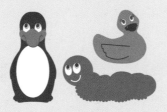

Novelty vibrators

Vibrators come in a vast number of cute or silly shapes, either to add a note of playfulness or to disguise their purpose. (Big Teaze Toys Penguin, Duckie, and

Basic massager

The simple, hard-plastic slim-line "massager" that was once the only easily obtainable sort of vibrator has been revived in a high-end version. (Jimmyjane Iconic

Waterproof slim-line

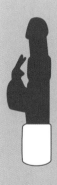

Able to be heated, cooled, or taken in the bath, this durable luxury vibrator comes in gold- and platinum-coated models; also available in even higher-end models, which are diamond embellished. (Jimmyjane Little Something)

Rabbit

This classic multitasker, made famous by the *Sex and the City* TV show, offers an insertable vibrator, rotating "pearls" for additional sensation, and a soft clitoral stimulator shaped like a little rabbit. Other models have various modifications. (Vibratex Rabbit Habit)

Bullet vibe

Small and discreet, the bullet vibe comes in a variety of colors and strengths. It can be used by itself, and many toys and strap-on harnesses have a small pouch that can fit one. (Hard Candy Bullet)

Couples' vibrator

Inserted before intercourse, this slim vibrator wraps around to stimulate the woman's G-spot and clitoris simultaneously and allows the man to share the vibrating sensation. (We-Vibe II)

Rechargeable G-spot vibrator

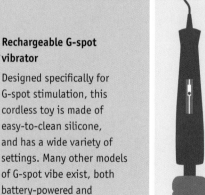

Designed specifically for G-spot stimulation, this cordless toy is made of easy-to-clean silicone, and has a wide variety of settings. Many other models of G-spot vibe exist, both battery-powered and plug-in. (LELO Gigi)

Wand-style vibrator

The large, soft head and easy-to-grip handle make this vibrator great for women who enjoy strong vibration. Attachments allow it to be used internally, and two women can use it for simultaneous clitoral stimulation. (Vibratex Hitachi Magic Wand)

Two-pronged vibrator

This high-end vibrator is waterproof, rechargeable, coated in silicone, and has dual motors, one in each prong. Other makers offer a number of variations. (Jimmyjane Form 2)

Oscillating vibrator

This versatile device oscillates instead of vibrating, and can be used with six different attachments for different sensations. (Eroscillator)

Wireless sound-activated vibrator

This toy offers the ability to switch from preprogrammed vibrating modes to one in which your MP3 player or home stereo controls the pulsing. (OhMiBod Freestyle)

Dual-stimulation vibrator

The "U" shape is designed to stimulate both the G-spot and the clitoris at the same time. (Natural Contours Ultime)

Prostate stimulator

Available in a range of sizes and subtle variations, these toys stimulate the prostate both internally and externally once fully inserted. (Aneros MGX)

Vibrating prostate stimulator

Some men find that the addition of vibration to prostate stimulation intensifies their experience. (Vibratex Pandora)

Egg

A stretchy silicone egg that is lubricated and placed over the head of the penis for masturbation. Available in a number of textures. (Tenga Egg)

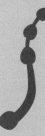

Stainless-steel beaded probe

This toy offers the popular beaded shape combined with steel's weight, and easy care. (njoy Fun Wand)

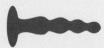

Silicone ripple plug

For those who enjoy a bit more texture, butt plugs can be purchased with ripples, beads, and other variations. The pleasure with these is often in slowly inserting or removing them so that the ripples can be felt. (Tantus Ripple)

Disposable sleeve

These moderately priced silicone-lined plastic sleeves are intended for a single use. Add-ons include lube and a "warming stick." (Tenga Onacup)

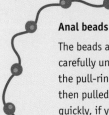

Anal beads

The beads are inserted carefully until nothing but the pull-ring remains, and then pulled out slowly—or quickly, if you prefer!

Flip hole

A high-tech masturbation aid with a multitexture silicone interior, hard case, and squeezable sides. The device can be opened for easy and thorough cleaning. (Tenga Flip Hole)

Silicone butt plug

Butt plugs come in an amazing array of sizes, shapes, and colors. The silicone ones are popular as they are firm yet yielding and easy to clean. (Tantus B-Bomb)

Stainless-steel butt plug

Available in a variety of shapes and sizes, these stainless steel plugs provide anal stimulation and are surprisingly heavy, which can intensify sensation. (njoy Pure Plug)

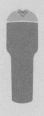

Fleshlight

The construction allows for hands-free operation—a man can prop this device in between couch cushions or under a mattress. (INL Fleshlight)

Double-ended dildo

These versatile toys can be shared by two partners of any gender or can be folded in half and used to double-penetrate a woman.

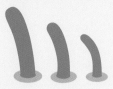

Nonrealistic dildo

In its simplest form, a "nonrealistic dildo" is anything that doesn't look like a penis. Smooth silicone dildos in a wide range of sizes are versatile and work well with a strap-on harness. (Tantus Silk)

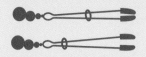

Tweezer clamps

Easily adjustable, these nipple clamps have soft rubber tips.

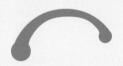

Stainless-steel G-spot wand

Made of metal, this toy holds heat or cold, is easy to clean, and, as a heavier insertable, provides slightly different sensation. (njoy Pure Wand)

Glass dildo

Some enjoy these for their beauty, others for the fact that they can be easily warmed or cooled and are easy to clean.

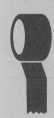

Bondage tape

Made of thin plastic, bondage tape sticks to itself, but not to skin, making it an easy way to restrain someone (or wrap a temporary outfit). It can easily be cut off with scissors and is reusable.

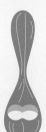

Wooden toys

Wood is warm and organic, but make sure that your wooden toys are finished with safe varnishes. (Nobessence Fling)

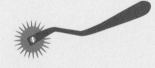

Wartenberg wheel

Originally designed to test nerve responses, it can be rolled gently or firmly over the body to produce sensations from tickling to pain.

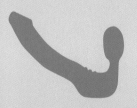

Hands-free double dildo

The "strapless strap-on" family of dildos is designed so that a woman can hold the bulb-shaped end inside her vagina or anus using only muscle power, and use the other end to penetrate a partner. Some models include a bullet vibe that stimulates partners on both ends of the toy. (Tantus Feeldoe)

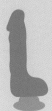

Realistic dildo

Anatomically-correct dildos come in a range of sizes. Some have suction cups for mounting (and mounting!) on hard surfaces.

Vibrating rings

Worn around the penis, these rings can have built-in vibrators or leave space for a bullet vibe. Either way, the vibrations add stimulation for the woman as well as pleasure for the man. (ScreamingO Vibrating Rings)

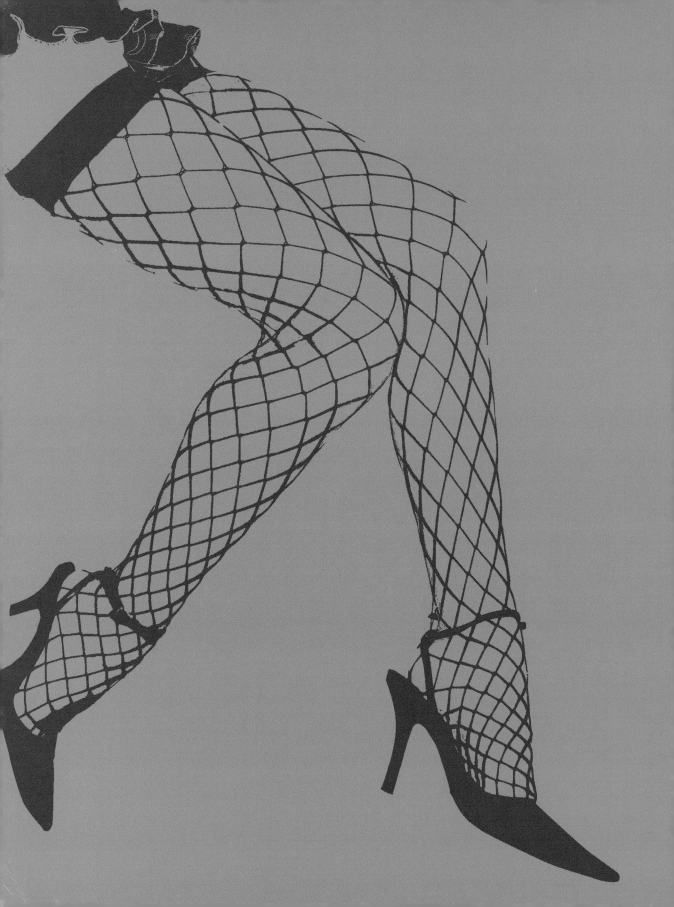

INDEX

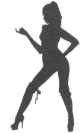

ABOUT THE AUTHORS

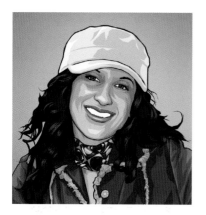

Jamye Waxman, M.Ed., holds a graduate degree in sex education from Philadelphia's Widener University. She is the former sex-advice columnist for *Playgirl* magazine and a writer for the *LA Weekly*'s After Dark. Jamye has also consulted for HBO's *The Katie Morgan Show,* and her work has appeared in *Women's Health, Men's Health, Zink, AVN Novelty, Xbiz, Steppin' Out,* and on Cherrytv.com, sexhealthguru.com, and RealitySandwich.com. The author of two prior books on sexuality, Jamye is also the creator and host of the *101 Positions for Lovers* and *Personal Touch* video series for Adam and Eve Pictures. She travels extensively teaching workshops on sexual pleasure and has been widely quoted in the media. The President of Feminists for Free Expression, she lives in Los Angeles and online at www.jamyewaxman.com.

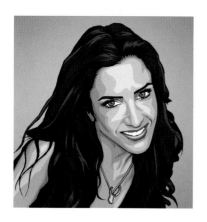

Emily Morse created the top-rated podcast "Sex with Emily" (www.sexwithemily.com), which is now a radio broadcast, as well as a popular iPhone app, "101 Sex Tips From Sex With Emily." She's syndicating the live radio show and has a television show in development. Emily has interviewed hundreds of experts about every realm of sexual experience, exploring topics from the common questions people ask to the outer realms of sexual exploration. She's been proud to welcome (and learn from) doctors, swingers, matchmakers, sex coaches, sensual-party hosts, sex-toy manufacturers, orgasmic monks, and many "real people," including happily married couples. Emily holds a degree in psychology from the University of Michigan, and has worked in documentary film and electoral politics in San Francisco.

ABOUT THE ILLUSTRATOR

Benjamin Wachenje started his career as a spray-can artist and went on to graduate in Fine Art and Graphic Design from Camberwell School of Arts. His illustrations continue to be influenced by the early hip-hop movement and contemporary street culture. His first solo exhibition, Open Mic (1997), was a series of portraits that documented underground British hip-hop artists. Since then he has been a contributor for numerous lifestyle magazines including *Wired, Stuff, ESPN,* and *Time,* as both an illustrator and graphic designer. Benjamin has been kept busy with mostly illustration and animation briefs and collaborations with advertising agencies. He has developed national campaigns for Timberland, British Telecom, BBC, MTV, Levi's, Nike, Toyota, Microsoft, Virgin Atlantic, SNCF, and Columbia Records. He lives and works in London.

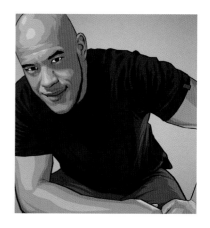

PANEL OF EXPERTS

Alan W. Shindel, M.D., completed his medical school and residency training in urology at Washington University in Saint Louis. He is currently a clinical instructor and fellow in andrology (men's reproductive and sexual health) at the University of California, San Francisco, and will be joining the faculty in the department of urology at the University of California, Davis, in August 2010. Dr. Shindel's clinical interests are the diagnosis and treatment of sexual disorders in both men and women; his research interests include sexuality education at the medical school level, sexual practices and function in sexual minority groups, alternative medical therapies for the treatment of sexual problems, and the basic science of sexual function.

Kathryn Ando holds a **Ph.D.** in Human Sexuality, and works with Project Prepare, an organization that teaches medical students at several prestigious universities (Stanford, Touro, and the University of California, San Francisco) about sexual health. She has coauthored papers related to sexual medicine as well as a book chapter on sex education for medical students. She is on the board of directors for the Center for Sex and Culture in San Francisco, which provides a library, media archive, and other resources to audiences across the sexual and gender spectrum.

Charlie Glickman, Ph.D., is the education-program manager at Good Vibrations, a leading sex-toy retail company and sexual-education hub. He holds a doctorate in Adult Sexuality Education from the Union Institute and University and is certified as a sexuality educator by the American Association of Sexuality Educators, Counselors, and Therapists. He has led workshops and done personal counseling on a broad range of sexuality-related topics, as well as adult education in other fields. He blogs regularly about sexuality, adult education, and culture at www.charlieglickman.com.

Toy Contributors

Thanks to the manufacturers who provided the following products for illustration:

FEATURED IN THE ACTIVITIES:

#13 **Sportsheets** Ostrich Tickler

#32 See Toy Glossary

#60 **Sportsheets** Under the Bed Restraint System

#74 **Tantus** Bend-Over-Beginner kit

FEATURED IN THE TOY GLOSSARY:

OhMiBod Club Vibe, Freestyle

Big Teaze Toys I Rub My Duckie, I Rub My Wormie, I Rub My Penguin

Jimmyjane Form 2, Iconic Smoothie, Little Something

Vibratex Hitachi Magic Wand, Pandora, Rabbit Habit, Water Dancer

LELO Gigi, Nea

Tenga Egg, Flip Hole, Onacup

njoy Fun Wand, Pure Plug, Pure Wand

Tantus B-bomb, Feeldoe, Ripple, Silk

NobEssence Inc. Fling

ScreamingO Vibrating rings, FingO Nubby

INL Fleshlight (courtesy of MyPleasure.com)

Aneros MGX

Advanced Response Corp. Eroscillator

Good Vibrations Hard Candy Bullet

We-Vibe We-Vibe II

Natural Contours Ultime

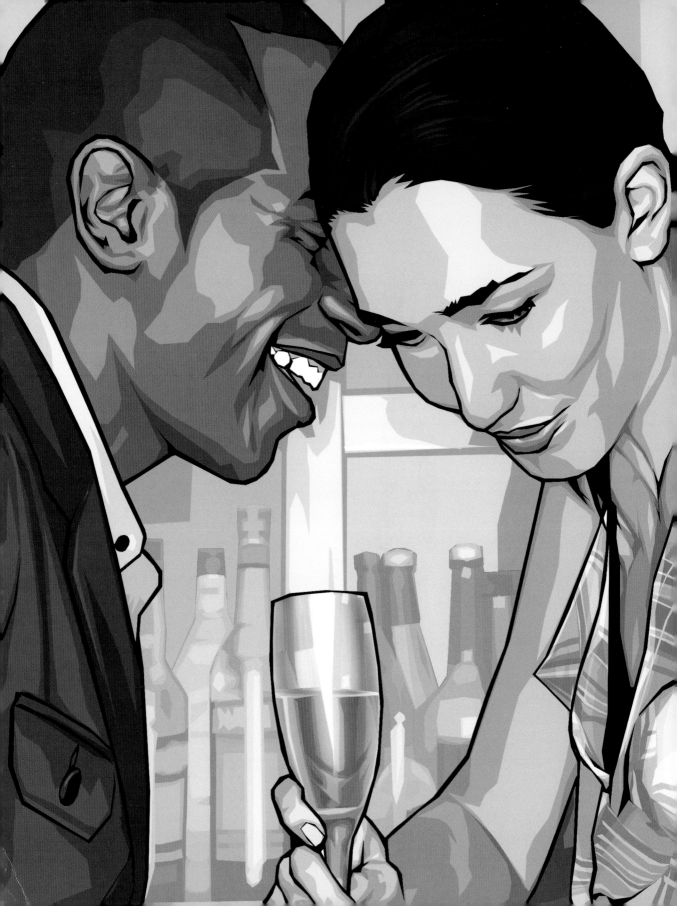

ACKNOWLEDGMENTS

Jamye Waxman

There are a lot of people to thank for so many things, but I'd like to acknowledge a few in my field and among my friends who have guided me to/through/during the writing of this book: Brooke Warner, Emily Morse, Candida Royalle, Ian and Alicia Denchasy, Barbara Carrellas, Paul Joannides, Cory Silverberg, Nina Hartley, Charlie Glickman, Mariah Bear, Nic Kazamia, Morty Diamond, Brian McCormack, Sasha Mazo, Jonathan Phillips, and Amy Rothlein Brown.

Also thanks to those who donated their fabulous products to these pages along with more fantastic and delightful sex educators, everyone at Weldon Owen, my family and friends.

Emily Morse

Thanks to the entire Weldon Owen crew, because, if you think sex is hard to talk about, try getting people to write a book about it. Special thanks to Roger for blushing your way through meetings, but still coming out in favor; and Mariah Bear, your growing enthusiasm made it all the more enjoyable.

Thanks to my coauthor Jamye—your words sparkle, as do you. Thanks to my mom for your steadfast support of my unconventional path. So many thanks to my friends for your wisdom and for always sharing your sexy secrets. Don't worry—I'll never tell. Thanks to Dr. Sandor Gardos from My Pleasure.com for all the sex toys you've gifted for "research," and for being a wonderful mentor and friend.

Thanks to all my listeners and guests of the "Sex With Emily" show who have taught me so much. We will continue to learn from each other. Finally, thanks in advance to my future lover for reading this book before we date. It'll save us some time.

Special thanks to the models who participated: Sara Bell, Barrie Evans, KayDee Kersten, Le'Evil, Winnie Leung, Madolyn McGuire MacKanin, Stephen Massey, Minx, Raz Neon, Simon Pearl, Space, Zev Ubu, and Scotch Wichmann.

Editorial expertise and assistance was provided by Maria Behan, Mikayla Butchart, Robert F. James, Marianna Monaco, Katharine Moore, Frances Reade, and Mary Zhang; design and photography support came from Conor Buckley, Hayden Foell, and Lisa Moir; research help by Sarah Lynn Duncan, Michael Alexander Eros, Sheila Masson, and Brandi Valenza. Many thanks to all.

Additional illustrations by Marisa Kwek.

weldonowen

415 Jackson Street
San Francisco, CA 94111
www.weldonowen.com

A division of
BONNIER

WELDON OWEN, INC.
President, CEO Terry Newell
VP, Sales Amy Kaneko
VP, Publisher Roger Shaw
Executive Editor Mariah Bear
Editor Lucie Parker
Editorial Assistant Emelie Griffin
Creative Director Kelly Booth
Art Director Marisa Kwek
Designer Meghan Hildebrand
Reference Photographers Delbarr Moradi, Erin Kunkel
Production Director Chris Hemesath
Production Manager Michelle Duggan
Color Manager Teri Bell

A WELDON OWEN PRODUCTION

© 2011 Weldon Owen Inc.

All rights reserved, including the right of reproduction in whole or in part in any form. Library of Congress Control Number on file with publisher.

ISBN 13: 978-1-61628-073-4
ISBN 10: 1-61628-073-5

10 9 8 7 6 5 4

2014 2013

Printed by Tien Wah Press in Singapore.

A Show Me Now Book.
Show Me Now is a trademark of Weldon Owen Inc.

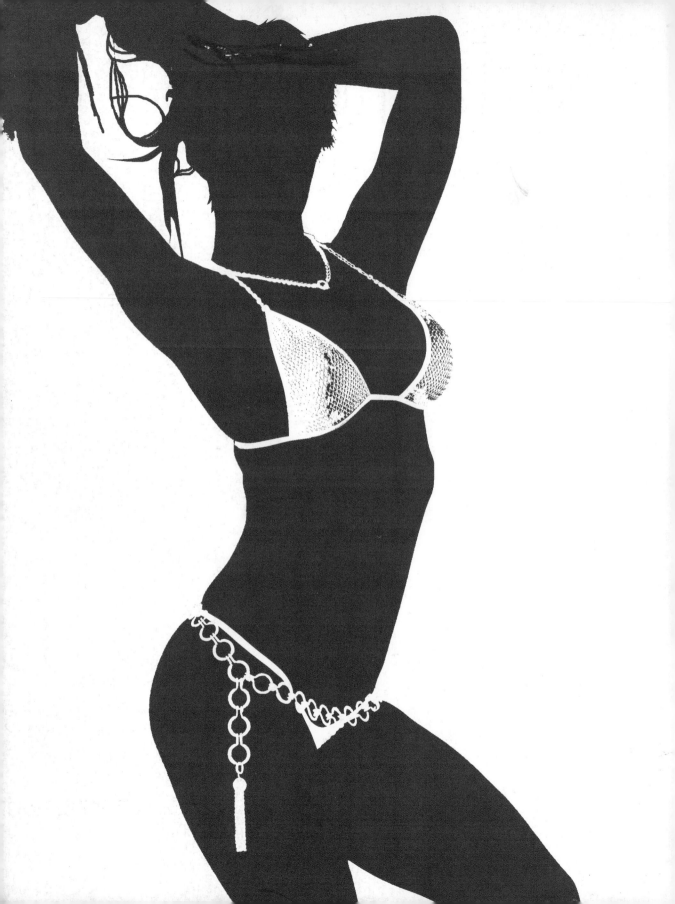